SWIMMING ANATOMY

ABERDEEN COLLEGE
GORDON LIBRARY

Ian McLeod

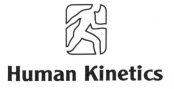

Human Kinetics

Library of Congress Cataloging-in-Publication Data

McLeod, Ian.
  Swimming anatomy / Ian McLeod.
     p. cm.
  ISBN-13: 978-0-7360-7571-8 (soft cover)
  ISBN-10: 0-7360-7571-2 (soft cover)
  1. Swimming--Training. 2. Swimming--Physiological aspects. 3. Aquatic sports injuries. I. Title.
  GV837.7.M37 2010
  797.2'1--dc22
                              2009016094

ISBN-10: 0-7360-7571-2 (print)   ISBN-10: 0-7360-8627-7 (Adobe PDF)
ISBN-13: 978-0-7360-7571-8 (print)   ISBN-13: 978-0-7360-8627-1 (Adobe PDF)

This publication is written and published to provide accurate and authoritative information relevant to the subject matter presented. It is published and sold with the understanding that the author and publisher are not engaged in rendering legal, medical, or other professional services by reason of their authorship or publication of this work. If medical or other expert assistance is required, the services of a competent professional person should be sought.

Acquisitions Editor: Tom Heine; **Developmental Editor:** Leigh Keylock; **Assistant Editor:** Laura Podeschi; **Copyeditor:** Bob Replinger; **Permission Manager:** Martha Gullo; **Graphic Designer:** Fred Starbird; **Graphic Artist:** Tara Welsch; **Cover Designer:** Keith Blomberg; **Photographer (for illustration references):** Neil Bernstein; **Photo Asset Manager:** Laura Fitch; **Visual Production Assistant:** Joyce Brumfield; **Art Manager:** Kelly Hendren; **Associate Art Manager:** Alan L. Wilborn; **Illustrator (cover):** Jennifer Gibas; **Illustrators (interior):** Jennifer Gibas and Becky Oles; **Printer:** United Graphics

Human Kinetics books are available at special discounts for bulk purchase. Special editions or book excerpts can also be created to specification. For details, contact the Special Sales Manager at Human Kinetics.

Printed in the United States of America   10 9 8 7 6 5 4 3 2

The paper in this book is certified under a sustainable forestry program.

Human Kinetics
Web site: www.HumanKinetics.com

United States: Human Kinetics
P.O. Box 5076
Champaign, IL 61825-5076
800-747-4457
e-mail: humank@hkusa.com

Canada: Human Kinetics
475 Devonshire Road, Unit 100
Windsor, ON N8Y 2L5
800-465-7301 (in Canada only)
e-mail: info@hkcanada.com

Europe: Human Kinetics
107 Bradford Road
Stanningley
Leeds LS28 6AT, United Kingdom
+44 (0)113 255 5665
e-mail: hk@hkeurope.com

Australia: Human Kinetics
57A Price Avenue
Lower Mitcham, South Australia 5062
08 8372 0999
e-mail: info@hkaustralia.com

New Zealand: Human Kinetics
P.O. Box 80
Torrens Park, South Australia 5062
0800 222 062
e-mail: info@hknewzealand.com

CONTENTS

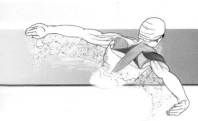

Swimming Anatomy is both a visual guide to the role of the musculoskeletal system in the four competitive swim strokes and a catalog of swimming-oriented dryland and weight-room exercises. The exercises in the text will help you maximize your performance and gain a competitive edge. Specific examples will help you choose exercises that target the most-used muscles for each stroke, starts, and turns to ensure that you are getting the best results from your program. Included are exercises that may help you prevent injuries by strengthening key stabilizing muscles and decreasing muscle imbalances. To help you understand how these exercises enhance performance, descriptions of the roles that various muscles play in propelling a swimmer through the water and guidance in using selected exercises to target those muscles are included. This chapter features an overview of the primary muscles used in the kicking motions and during the pull-through and recovery phases of freestyle, butterfly, backstroke, and breaststroke. The chapter also addresses some strength and conditioning principles and how they relate to designing a swimming-specific dryland program. Chapters 2 through 8, organized according to major body parts, each contain exercises with accompanying illustrations and easy-to-follow descriptions and instructions. The anatomical illustrations that accompany the exercises are color-coded to indicate the primary and secondary muscles and connective tissues featured in each exercise and swimming-specific movement.

■ Primary muscles	▦ Secondary muscles	☐ Connective tissues

Swimmers face several unique challenges that athletes in most land-based sports do not encounter. The first challenge is the total-body nature of all four competitive strokes, which involve movements of both the upper and lower extremities. A coordinated effort of the musculoskeletal system is required to keep each body part moving correctly to maximize efficiency of movement through the water. To visualize this coordinated effort, think of the body as a long chain and each body segment as a link in the chain. Because all the segments are linked together, movement in one segment affects all the other segments. This linkage, commonly referred to as the kinetic chain, allows the power generated by the arms to be transferred through the torso to the legs. But if a link in the chain is weak, a loss of power transfer can occur, bodily movements can become uncoordinated, and the risk of injury can increase.

Another unique demand of swimming is that swimmers are required to create their own base of support. Unlike land-based athletes, who have a stable surface to push off from, you have to generate your own base of support, because most training takes place in a fluid environment. The key to linking the movement of the upper and lower extremities in the water, and at the same time generating a firm base of support, is a strong and stable core. The core is best thought of as the foundation on which the muscles of the upper and lower body are built. Even a strong and well-designed house will eventually deteriorate if the foundation is weak.

Without a doubt, swimming itself is the most effective way to become a better and faster swimmer, but several components outside the water play an important role in how you develop as a swimmer. One of those is a well-designed dryland program based on an appreciation of the relationship between the body's muscular framework and stroke mechanics. While engaged in swimming, muscles primarily function as either the mover of a body segment or a stabilizer of a body segment. An example of a muscle functioning as a mover is the latissimus dorsi, commonly known as the lats, moving the arm through the water during the propulsive phase of all four competitive strokes. The near-constant activity of the core abdominal musculature is a prime example of a group of muscles functioning as a stabilizing mechanism. Both functions are vital to proper stroke mechanics and efficient movement through the water. Descriptions of the muscle recruitment patterns for each of the four strokes are categorized as those that are active during the propulsive phase, the recovery phase, and kicking.

 freestyle

 backstroke

 breaststroke

 butterfly

 starts and turns

Throughout the exercise descriptions in the subsequent chapters you will see a series of five icons, one for each of the strokes and one for starts and turns. The purpose of these icons is to identify the exercises that are particularly well suited to a specific stroke or starts and turns.

Freestyle

As the hand enters into the water, the wrist and elbow follow and the arm is extended to the starting position of the propulsive phase. Upward rotation of the shoulder blade allows the swimmer to reach an elongated position in the water. From this elongated position, the first part of the propulsive phase begins with the catch. The initial movements are first generated by the clavicular portion of the pectoralis major. The latissimus dorsi quickly joins in to assist the pectoralis major. These two muscles generate a majority of the force during the underwater pull, mostly during the second half of the pull. The wrist flexors act to hold the wrist in a position of slight flexion for the entire duration of the propulsive phase. At the elbow, the elbow flexors (biceps brachii and brachialis) begin to contract at the start of the catch phase, gradually taking the elbow from full extension into approximately 30 degrees of flexion.

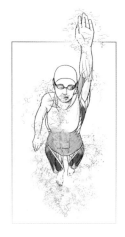

During the final portion of the propulsive phase the triceps brachii acts to extend the elbow, which brings the hand backward and upward toward the surface of the water, thus ending the propulsive phase. The total amount of extension taking place depends on your specific stroke mechanics and the point at which you initiate your recovery. The deltoid and rotator cuff (supraspinatus, infraspinatus, teres minor, and subscapularis) are the primary muscles active during the recovery phase, functioning to bring the arm and hand out of the water near the hips and return them to an overhead position for reentry into the water. The arm movements during freestyle are reciprocal in nature, meaning that while one arm is engaged in propulsion, the other is in the recovery process.

Several muscle groups function as stabilizers during both the propulsive phase and the recovery phase. One of the key groups is the shoulder blade stabilizers (pectoralis minor, rhomboid, levator scapula, middle and lower trapezius, and the serratus anterior), which as the name implies serve to anchor or stabilize the shoulder blade. Proper functioning of this muscle group is important because all the propulsive forces generated by the arm and hand rely on the scapula's having a firm base of support. Additionally, the shoulder blade stabilizers work with the deltoid and rotator cuff to reposition the arm during the recovery phase. The core stabilizers (transversus abdominis, rectus abdominis, internal oblique, external oblique, and erector spinae) are also integral to efficient stroke mechanics because they serve as a link between the movements of the upper and lower extremities. This link is central to coordination of the body roll that takes place during freestyle swimming.

Like the arm movements, the kicking movements can be categorized as a propulsive phase and a recovery phase; these are also referred to as the downbeat and the upbeat. The propulsive phase (downbeat) begins at the hips by activation of the iliopsoas and rectus femoris muscles. The rectus femoris also initiates extension of the knee, which follows shortly after hip flexion begins. The quadriceps (vastus lateralis, vastus intermedius, and vastus medialis) join the rectus femoris to help generate more forceful extension of the knee. Like the propulsive phase, the recovery phase starts at the hips with contraction of the gluteal muscles (primarily gluteus maximus and medius) and is quickly followed by contraction of the hamstrings (biceps femoris, semitendinosus, and semimembranosus). Both muscle groups function as hip extensors. Throughout the entire kicking motion the foot is maintained in a plantarflexed position secondary to activation of the gastrocnemius and soleus and pressure exerted by the water during the downbeat portion of the kick.

Butterfly

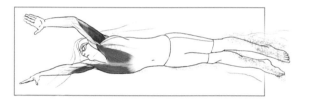

The primary difference between freestyle and butterfly is that the arms move in unison during butterfly whereas reciprocal movements take place with freestyle. Because butterfly and freestyle have the same underwater pull pattern, the muscle recruitment patterns are almost identical. As with freestyle, the swimmer's arms in butterfly are in an elongated position when they initiate the propulsive underwater portion of the stroke. Muscles active during the entire propulsive phase are the pectoralis major and latissimus dorsi, which function as the primary movers, and the wrist flexors, which act to maintain the wrist in a neutral to slightly flexed position. The biceps brachii and brachialis are active as the elbow moves from being fully extended at the initiation of the catch to approximately 40 degrees of flexion during the midpart of the pull. Unlike in freestyle, a forceful extension of the elbow is emphasized during the final portion of the pull, resulting in greater demands being placed on the triceps brachii. As in the freestyle stroke, both the rotator cuff and deltoid are responsible for moving the arm during the recovery phase, but the mechanics are somewhat different. Butterfly lacks the body roll that aids the recovery process during freestyle; instead, an undulating movement of the torso occurs, which brings the entire upper torso out of the water to aid in the recovery process.

Again, the shoulder blade stabilizing muscles are extremely important, because they function to provide a firm anchor point for the propulsive forces generated by the arms and help reposition the arms during the recovery phase of the stroke. Although butterfly lacks the body roll present in freestyle, the core stabilizers are still important in linking the movements of the upper and lower extremities and have an important role in creating the undulating motion that allows the swimmer to get the upper torso and arms out of the water during the recovery process. The undulating movement is initiated with contraction of the paraspinal muscles that run in multiple groups from the lower portion of the back to the base of the skull. This contraction results in an arching of the back, at which time the arms are moving through the recovery process. Contraction of the abdominal muscles quickly follows, which prepares the upper body to follow the entry of the hands into the water to initiate the propulsive phase of the stroke.

As with the arms, the muscles used in generating the kicking movements during the butterfly kick are identical to those used during the freestyle kick; the only difference in kick mechanics is that the legs move in unison. The propulsive downbeat begins with contraction of the iliopsoas and rectus femoris, acting as hip flexors. The rectus femoris also initiates knee extension, and associated firing of the quadriceps muscle group further aids in extension of the knee. The gluteal muscle group drives the recovery phase of the kick. Concomitant contraction of the hamstring muscles also works to extend the hip. The foot is maintained in a plantarflexed position through a combination of the resistance from the water and activation of the gastrocnemius and soleus, acting as plantarflexors. The dolphin kick that is used at the start of the race and off each turn wall recruits a larger group of muscles than the smaller, more isolated kick tied into the arm movements. Besides the movements generated at the hips and knee, the dolphin kick ties in the undulating movements of the torso through activation of the core stabilizers and the paraspinal musculature.

Backstroke

Although backstroke is unique in body positioning among the competitive strokes, the stroke phases can still be divided into a propulsive phase that consists of hand entry into the water, a catch component, a finishing component, and a recovery phase. Rotation at the shoulder puts the hands in a position in which the little finger is the first to enter the water. Combined with extension of the elbow, the swimmer is in an elongated position to begin the underwater propulsion phase of the stroke. A difference between backstroke and freestyle or butterfly is that the initial catch component is

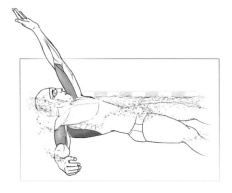

dominated by the latissimus dorsi. The pectoralis major makes a smaller contribution. Despite these differences the latissimus dorsi and the pectoralis major are still the prime movers and are active to some degree throughout the entire propulsive phase. Although the wrist flexors are still an integral part of the entire propulsion phase, the wrist is maintained in a neutral to slightly extended position. Through a combination of pressure forces from the water and activation of the biceps brachii and brachialis, the elbow transitions into approximately 45 degrees of flexion at the start of the catch. By the end of the catch the elbow may be flexed as much as 90 degrees just before transitioning into the finishing component. As with the finishing component in butterfly, more emphasis is placed on forceful extension of the elbow, placing high demand on the triceps brachii during the final portion of the propulsive phase.

The role of the stabilizing musculature during backstroke is similar to the role that it plays in freestyle, largely because of the similar reciprocal arm movement and the integration of body roll into both strokes.

The kicking motion seen in backstroke is a combination of movements that we have seen in freestyle and butterfly kicking mechanics. Like freestyle, backstroke uses reciprocal kicking movements. The major difference is that the position of the swimmer causes most of the force to be generated during the upbeat portion of the kick as opposed to the downbeat in freestyle. Backstroke also uses the dolphin kick off the start of a race and off each wall. The muscle recruitment patterns are the same in each case; the only change is in the direction because of the swimmer's body position.

Breaststroke

As with the other strokes the arm movements that take place during breaststroke are categorized as a propulsive phase and a recovery phase. The propulsive phase begins with the shoulders and arms in an elongated overhead position. The first half of the underwater pull is similar to that used in freestyle and butterfly. The clavicular portion of the pectoralis major starts the movement, and the latissimus dorsi quickly joins in. During the second half of the pull, forceful contractions of the pectoralis major and latissimus dorsi pull the arms and hands into the midline of the body to finish the pull. The forces generated during the final phase are directed toward forward propulsion of the swimmer in the water and upward propulsion of the swimmer's torso, which is aided by contraction of the paraspinal muscles. This movement brings the swimmer's head and shoulders out of the water. Flexion and rotation at the elbow 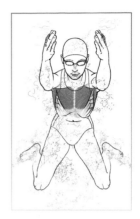 bring the hands to the midline of the body and mark the conversion into the recovery phase. To return the hands to the starting position, the arms must be returned from their position under the chest. This motion is carried out by recruitment of the pectoralis major, anterior deltoid, and the long head of the biceps brachii, which all function to flex the shoulder joint. At the same time, extension of the elbow by the triceps brachii results in completion of the recovery phase, and the arms return to their extended and elongated position.

As with the other strokes, the shoulder blade stabilizing musculature is crucial to creating a firm base of support for the movements and forces generated by the arms. Like the butterfly stroke, the breaststroke lacks a body roll component. Even so, the core-stabilizing musculature is important in ensuring an efficient linkage between the movement patterns of the upper and lower extremities.

Like the arm movements, the kicking mechanics can be divided into a propulsive phase, consisting of outsweep and insweep components, and a recovery phase. The propulsive phase begins with the feet hip-width apart and the knees and hips in a flexed position. The outsweep is initiated with outward rotation of the feet, which is accomplished by a combination of movements at the hip, knee, and ankle. After the foot has been turned outward, the outer sweeping motion is continued by extension of the hip and knee. The gluteal musculature and the hamstrings function to extend the hip, and the rectus femoris and quadriceps act to straighten the knee. At the transition from the outsweep to the insweep, the knees and hip are still not completely extended, so the respective muscle groups continue their action into the insweep component until the knees and hip are fully extended. At the start of the insweep the legs are in an abducted position, generating an opportunity for force production through rapid adduction of the legs. The legs are brought back together by contraction of the adductor muscles that run along the upper portion of the inner thigh. To minimize drag during the final portion of the insweep, the calf muscles are activated to bring the foot and ankle into a pointed position. Recovery is accomplished by recruitment of the rectus femoris and iliopsoas, which serve to flex the hip, and recruitment of the hamstrings, which serve to flex the knee.

Dryland Training Programs

Although this book is not intended to give full program design details and guidelines, it does provide you with an understanding of how each exercise can directly benefit you as a swimmer, which in turn can help you make better decisions when choosing exercises for a specific program design. For example, if your program calls for an exercise that targets the triceps, you have many to choose from in chapter 2. We will, however, lay out some general principles and ideas for training programs here.

You should be aware of several considerations when designing a dryland program. The repetitive nature of swimming predisposes swimmers to developing muscle imbalances. Muscles such as the latissimus dorsi and pectoralis major become overdeveloped in relation to the smaller muscles that make up the scapular stabilizers (particularly the middle and lower trapezius and the rhomboids). In the lower extremity the quadriceps and hip flexors often become dominant over weaker hamstrings and gluteal muscles. These muscle imbalances not only lead to strength imbalances but also may create flexibility and postural imbalances that can predispose you to injury and inhibit optimal performance. So when designing a dryland program you should include a flexibility component. Recent findings in the realm of flexibility training are that dynamic stretches and movement patterns are an effective way to prepare for an exercise session. Dynamic movements and stretches can be designed to incorporate whole-body movements that can serve as an effective low-intensity warm-up while also addressing areas of inflexibility. Further attention can be given to tight muscle groups through static stretching at the conclusion of the dryland program.

Careful consideration needs to be given to selecting the proper exercises. Two concepts that can help guide exercise choice are transference and isolation. Transference is the ability of an exercise to strengthen muscles in a manner that will benefit a certain skill or task, in this case swimming. Transference can be further divided into direct and indirect forms. Direct transference involves choosing an exercise because the associated movements are directly related to a certain component of one of the major strokes. An example would be using the physioball prone streamline exercise (see page 136), because it directly mimics the streamlined position that swimmers hold off their starts and walls. Indirect transference involves choosing a certain exercise because the targeted muscle groups are similar to those used during a phase of one of the major strokes or choosing a certain exercise because it can transfer to a certain stroke component. An example would be selecting the lat pull-down exercise (see page 120) because it targets the latissimus dorsi muscle, which is a prime mover of the arms in each of the major strokes. Isolation involves choosing an exercise that emphasizes a certain muscle or muscle group with the goal of strengthening an area that (1) may be underdeveloped because of muscle imbalances, (2) is important for injury prevention, or (3) has been identified as an area of weakness by something in the swimmer's stroke profile.

Another choice concerns which model of dryland training to use—a traditional weight-training program or a circuit-based program. Traditional weight-training programs involve performing a certain number of sets and repetitions of one or two exercises at a time and then moving on to the next set of exercises. These programs are better reserved for swimmers near college age and older. In contrast, circuit-training programs involve a series of exercises performed one after another. After performing one set of an exercise, the person moves on to the next. Circuit programs are ideal when (1) the dryland program is being performed on a pool deck, (2) a large group of swimmers is participating in the program at the same time, or (3) a younger group of swimmers is training. An additional advantage of circuit programs is that they are time efficient, allowing a large number of exercises to be completed in a short time.

To maximize your gains when performing a traditional or circuit dryland program, give careful attention to the order in which you perform the exercises. All programs should begin with a 10-minute warm-up period consisting of dynamic flexibility exercises and low-intensity aerobics. Following the warm-up, you should incorporate several injury prevention and core stabilization exercises (choose from those in chapter 5). You should begin with total-body exercises that combine movements of the upper and lower extremities and progress to multijoint exercises and then isolation exercises. For example, when training the upper extremity and shoulder girdle, you could begin with a single-arm lawn mower (page 176), follow with a barbell flat bench press (page 70), and end with a dumbbell biceps curl (page 28). The underlying concept is to avoid performing the biceps curl first, which would fatigue the biceps brachii and decrease the overall weight that you could lift with the single-arm lawn mower exercise. A swimming analogy would be to avoid performing an exhaustive kick set before you perform your main quality freestyle set during a workout, because fatiguing your legs would limit your ability to get the full benefit from the freestyle set. Following completion of the main exercises, you can spend time on additional core stabilization exercises and static stretching and flexibility. Note that your final program should consist of more than three exercises; the limited number used in this case serve only as an example.

Another concept to consider is that of pushing and pulling exercises. Pushing exercises such as push-ups and bench presses primarily work the pectoral muscles and the triceps, whereas pulling exercises such as pull-ups and seated rows primarily work the lats and biceps. Because these types of exercises mirror each other in the muscle groups that they target, doing one after the other is often beneficial in a dryland program because the alternating nature of exercises allows one group to recover while the other is being exercised.

The next question to address is how many sets and repetitions of each exercise you should perform. The number of repetitions is dictated by the inverse relationship between volume and intensity. Exercise volume is equal to the total number of repetitions performed, and intensity is a measure of the effort being exerted when performing a given exercise. What this means is that as you increase the number of repetitions of a given exercise, the overall intensity at which you will be able to perform that exercise will decrease. For example, you may be able to perform 15 dumbbell kickbacks with 25 pounds (11 kg), but if you were to pick up a 40-pound (18 kg) dumbbell, you might be able to perform only 8 repetitions. This relationship becomes important, depending on your training goal. If you are trying to improve muscular endurance, you should choose a weight that allows you to perform 15 to 20 repetitions. If your goal is to build strength, you should use a weight that allows you to perform only 5 to 8 repetitions. Generally, when performing more repetitions (15 to 20) you should perform two sets, whereas when you are doing fewer repetitions (5 to 8) you should perform four or five sets. Your combination of sets and repetitions is probably appropriate for a given exercise if the targeted muscles feel fatigued during the last 2 to 3 repetitions of the final set. With circuit-training programs, the number of repetitions can be either predetermined or time dependent. For example, at one station you might perform 30 sit-ups (set number of reps) or as many sit-ups as you can in one minute (time dependent).

Your training goal in regard to endurance versus strength will depend on where you are in the season. The principle of periodization comes into play here. Periodization involves breaking the season into various phases, each with a different training goal. The underlying purpose is to prevent overtraining and maximize performance.

Dryland Training for Young Swimmers

An important consideration in training is the age of the swimmer. Not too long ago, strength, or resistance, training was considered inappropriate and potentially dangerous to the young athlete. Participation in resistance training was thought to increase the risk of injury to the growth plate, which could have negative consequences to the child's growth. But the safety and effectiveness of resistance training in youth is now well documented and supported by position or policy statements from the American College of Sports Medicine (ACSM), American Academy of Pediatrics (AAP), American Orthopaedic Society for Sports Medicine (AOSSM), and the National Strength and Conditioning Association (NSCA).

Resistance training helps young swimmers develop an enjoyable and positive outlook by increasing their chance of success through improved performance and decreasing their risk of injury. With a focus on fundamental fitness ability, resistance training also prepares them for the demands of in-water practices. Specific benefits may include improvements in muscular power, muscular endurance, total body strength, stability around joints, body composition, and bone mineral density, all of which can improve sport performance.

The research indicates that training-induced strength gains during preadolescence are possible if the training program is of sufficient duration, intensity, and volume. Current recommendations are that to produce strength gains, young athletes should perform two or three sets of 13 to 15 repetitions for each exercise. Training sessions should take place two to three days per week on nonconsecutive days. Note that these gains often result from adaptations in neuromuscular factors such as motor unit activation, recruitment, and coordination rather than increased muscle size (hypertrophy). Younger athletes do not have enough muscle-building hormones to cause muscle hypertrophy, but following puberty, training-induced gains in males and females are associated with increased muscle mass because of hormonal influences. Resistance training will not lead to increases in height, but no data indicate that training will stunt skeletal growth.

Before a young swimmer begins a resistance program, he or she should have sufficient emotional maturity to accept and follow directions. The athlete should also be able to understand the benefits and risks associated with a resistance-training program and specific exercises. When selecting exercises keep in mind that swimmers in a given age range can vary significantly in strength and coordination. Exercises should be selected on an individual basis and modified if necessary. Guidelines are provided throughout the text about exercises that may not be suitable for young swimmers, and examples are offered about how to modify exercises to make them more age appropriate.

When designing resistance-training programs for young athletes, a progressive and step-wise approach in exercise prescription is recommended. This approach stresses proper form and technique, adequate supervision of all training sessions, and a slow, stepwise progression of exercises. Kraemer and Fleck (2005) illustrate the importance of proper exercise selection and considerations for athletes of various ages (table 1.1).

When considering the important role of each muscle in the mechanics of the four swim strokes, you can see that keeping the muscles strong and well conditioned is critical to maintaining proper technique, improving performance, and minimizing risk of injury. Each of the following chapters includes exercises that target various muscles in a manner that contributes directly to swim-specific movements.

Table 1.1   Age-Related Resistance-Training Considerations

Ages	Considerations
7 and younger	Introduce child to basic exercises with little or no weight; develop the concept of a training session; teach technique; progress from bodyweight calisthenics, partner exercises, and light resistance; keep volume low.
8–10	Gradually increase the number of exercises; practice technique on all lifts; start gradual progressive loading; keep exercises simple; gradually increase volume; carefully monitor toleration to exercise stress.
11–13	Teach all basic exercise techniques; continue progressive loading of each exercise; emphasize technique; introduce more advanced exercises with little or no resistance; increase volume.
14–15	Progress to more advanced youth programs in resistance exercise; add sport-specific components; emphasize techniques; increase volume.
16 and older	Move child to entry-level adult programs after all background knowledge has been mastered and a basic level of training experience has been gained.

Adapted, by permission, from W.J. Kraemer and S.J. Fleck, 2005, *Strength training for young athletes,* 2nd ed. (Champaign, IL: Human Kinetics), 13.

CHAPTER 2

The arms are extremely important in swimming because they are the link between the primary force-generating muscles of the upper extremity, the latissimus dorsi and pectoralis major, and the hands and forearms, which are the anchor points that propel the swimmer through the water. Chapter 1 compared the body to a chain that starts at the hands and extends all the way down to the feet. The main point was that, as a swimmer moves through the water, movements and forces are transmitted along the chain and that the chain is only as strong as its weakest link. Of course, the arm muscles also aid in generating the forces that propel you through the water. Those reasons should help you understand the importance of targeting the arm muscles with a dryland program.

The elbow divides the arm into an upper and lower component. The elbow is a hinge joint restricted to two movements, extension and flexion. Elbow extension occurs when you straighten your arm, moving the forearm away from the upper arm. Elbow flexion is the opposite, involving bending the forearm toward the upper arm. The structural framework of the upper arm is the humerus. The lower arm, typically called the forearm (figure 2.1, *a-b*), is supported by the radius and ulna. These three bones are the major attachment sites and

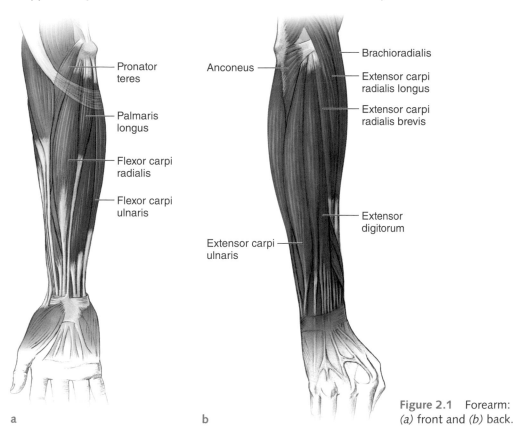

Pronator teres

Palmaris longus

Flexor carpi radialis

Flexor carpi ulnaris

Anconeus

Extensor carpi ulnaris

Brachioradialis

Extensor carpi radialis longus

Extensor carpi radialis brevis

Extensor digitorum

Figure 2.1 Forearm: (*a*) front and (*b*) back.

a

b

levers upon which the muscles of the arm and forearm originate and act on. The two primary muscle groups in the arms that are the target of the strengthening exercises in this chapter are the elbow extensors and elbow flexors. Both contribute to the maintenance of proper arm position and propulsion during each of the four competitive strokes.

The primary elbow extensor is the triceps brachii (figure 2.2). *Triceps* refers to its three heads of proximal attachment, and *brachii* refers to its origination in the arm. The medial and lateral heads arise from attachment sites on the humerus, and the long head crosses the shoulder joint and arises from the scapula (shoulder blade). The three heads unite to form the tendon that crosses behind the elbow joint and inserts onto the olecranon process of the ulna. The olecranon process forms the tip of the elbow when it is bent to 90 degrees. A much smaller triangular muscle called the anconeus assists the triceps in extending the elbow joint and is important as an elbow stabilizer. The anconeus is intimate with the lateral head of the triceps brachii; sometimes the fibers of the two muscles blend into one another.

The primary elbow flexors are the biceps brachii and the brachialis (figure 2.3). As the name implies, the biceps has two heads, a long and a short, both of which cross the shoulder joint and attach to the scapula. The two heads fuse to form a common tendon that crosses the front of the elbow joint to attach to the radius approximately 1.5 inches (4 cm) past the elbow. Besides being an elbow flexor, the biceps brachii contributes to the forearm movement of supination, which is the position when the palm is facing up. Your hands would be in this position to carry a bowl of soup. The brachialis lies beneath the biceps brachii and arises at the midpoint of the humerus. It attaches to the ulna just after it passes anteriorly to (in front of) the elbow joint. A smaller muscle that at times contributes to elbow flexion is the brachioradialis. This muscle arises from the lateral aspect of the humerus just above the elbow and travels along the outer part of the forearm to attach to the radius just above the wrist joint.

Despite difference in stroke mechanics, freestyle, butterfly, and backstroke have similar activation patterns of the elbow flexors and extensors during the pull phase. As the swim-

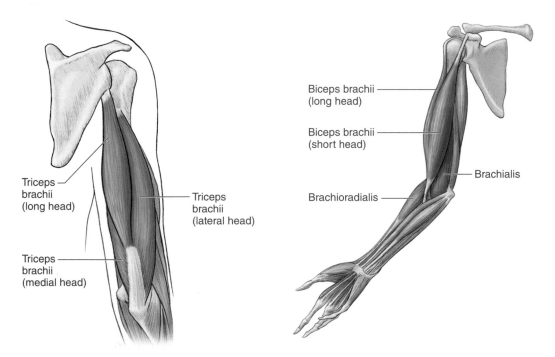

Figure 2.2   Triceps brachii.

Figure 2.3   Biceps brachii, brachialis, and brachioradialis.

mer progresses through the catch, the elbow moves from full extension to a position of 30 to 90 degrees of elbow flexion at midpull, depending on the stroke and the swimmer's mechanics. The primary muscles responsible for generating the change in elbow position and, when necessary, maintaining the elbow in a fixed position of flexion are the biceps brachii and brachialis. After the elbow reaches a point of maximal flexion during the midpull, it progresses into an extended position during the remainder of the pull phase. This action aids in generating propulsive forces and is brought about primarily by active recruitment of the triceps brachii. The degree of the propulsive force generated depends on the point in the pull phase at which the swimmer removes the hand from the water to initiate the recovery phase. In freestyle and butterfly many coaches are now teaching their swimmers to begin the recovery process as the hand reaches the hip, before the elbow is fully extended. Meanwhile, backstroke mechanics involve the catch phase, terminating with full extension of the elbow joint.

Unlike in the other strokes, during the initial portion of the pull phase of the breaststroke the triceps brachii is the primary muscle that is active at the elbow joint, functioning to maintain the elbow in a position near full extension. As the hands begin to turn inward marking the transition from the outsweep to the insweep, the muscle activation patterns at the elbow begin to change. The elbow flexors (biceps brachii and brachialis) activate to bring the elbow into a flexed position, a movement that aids in the generation of propulsive force. As the swimmer transitions into the recovery phase, the recruitment pattern changes again. The triceps brachii becomes activated to extend the elbow joint, thereby straightening the arm and preparing the swimmer to begin the next pull phase.

As you read through the remainder of the chapter you will see that several of the exercises involve movement at a single joint, the elbow, specifically targeting only the elbow extensors (triceps brachii) or the elbow flexors (biceps brachii and brachialis). These isolation exercises are best placed at the end of your dryland program to avoid fatiguing a single muscle group early in the workout program. A final consideration is that between the two muscle groups, the elbow extensors are more active during the swimming movements. Therefore, you should aim for a 2:1 ratio between exercises that target the extensors and the flexors.

When performing upper-body exercises, be sure to set the shoulder blades for stability before performing the exercise. For any exercise, set the core as well. See the sidebar below for instructions about how to do this.

Setting the Shoulder Blades and the Core

Setting the shoulder blades: When performing upper-extremity exercises, particularly those that target the shoulder joint, you should set the shoulder blades into a stable position. The setting movement involves pinching the shoulder blades backward and downward, as if you were trying to put your shoulder blades in the back pockets of your pants. In the process of setting the shoulder blades, avoid shrugging the shoulders upward because this action shifts the focus of the exercise from the lower fibers of the trapezius muscle to the upper fibers, which are typically already overdeveloped in most swimmers.

Setting the core: Before performing any exercise you should make a conscious effort to set the core. By setting the core you establish a foundation of support upon which the exercising muscles are able to exert their forces. You should also stabilize the low back, reducing the risk of injury. Setting the core involves simultaneously contracting the abdominal, low back, and gluteal muscles as if they are a corset that encircles the abdominal region. See chapter 5, page 87, for more information about setting the core.

Standing Double-Arm Triceps Pushdown

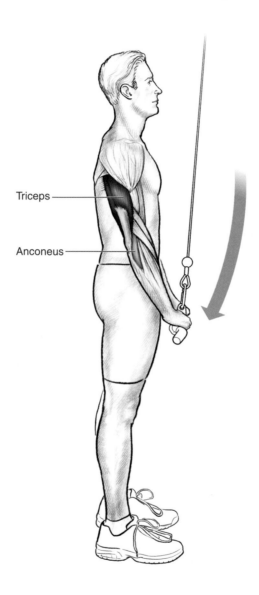

Triceps

Anconeus

Execution

1. Stand facing a pulley machine with a high cable attachment. Grasp the handlebar at chest level using an overhand grip so that your hands are slightly less than shoulder-width apart.

2. Holding your elbows tight at your sides, extend the forearms until the elbows are almost locked.

3. Slowly lower the weight stack until it is 1 inch (2.5 cm) above the resting stack and your hands are back to the start position.

Muscles Involved

Primary: Triceps brachii

Secondary: Anconeus, wrist and finger flexors

Swimming Focus

Although this exercise is effective at targeting the triceps brachii and will produce benefits across all four strokes, it is particularly valuable to breaststrokers because it mimics the final portion of the underwater pull performed off the start and each turn wall.

When performing the exercise you should maintain an upright posture and try to generate the force necessary to move the weight solely by tightening your triceps brachii. Because swimmers have a predisposition to a rounded-shoulder posture, you can easily develop the bad habit of leaning into the cable and cheating by bouncing your upper body at the start of each repetition.

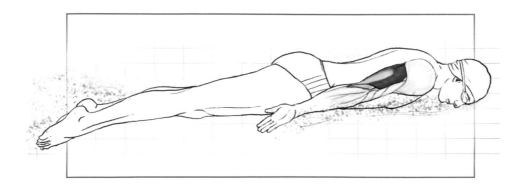

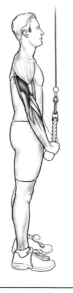

VARIATION

Standing Double-Arm Triceps Pushdown With Rope

In the starting position your hands are at your midline. As the elbows are extended, the hands pull the ends of the ropes outward so that when the elbows are almost locked the hands are shoulder-width apart. The added lateral movement isolates the lateral head of the triceps brachii.

Dumbbell Kickback

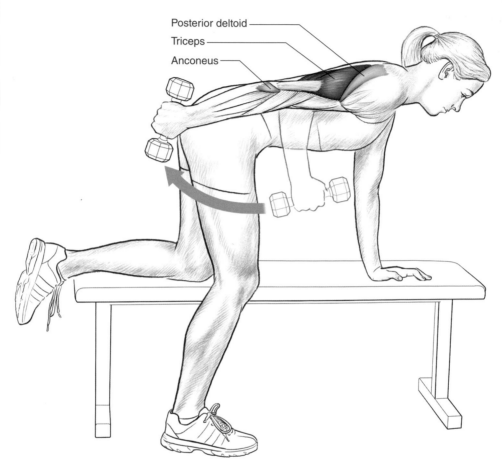

Posterior deltoid
Triceps
Anconeus

Execution

1. Holding a dumbbell in one hand, support your upper body with your free hand and a knee on an exercise bench.
2. With your upper arm parallel to the floor and your forearm vertical, raise the dumbbell upward until the elbow is almost locked.
3. Lower the dumbbell back to the 90-degree bent-elbow position.

Muscles Involved

Primary: Triceps brachii

Secondary: Posterior deltoid, latissimus dorsi, anconeus, wrist and finger flexors

Swimming Focus

Dumbbell kickbacks help strengthen the triceps brachii because they move the elbow through the final 90 degrees of extension, an important range when trying to enhance the propulsive forces generated during the final portion of the pull during freestyle, butterfly, and especially backstroke.

Slow, controlled movements are the key to maximizing the benefits of this exercise. The best way to enforce this is to pause for one to two seconds when the arm is fully extended, with a focus on squeezing the triceps tight, and to pause for one to two seconds when the arm is in the 90-degree bent-elbow position. This approach will prevent you from generating a pendulum-like swinging motion with the dumbbell, which is a form of cheating.

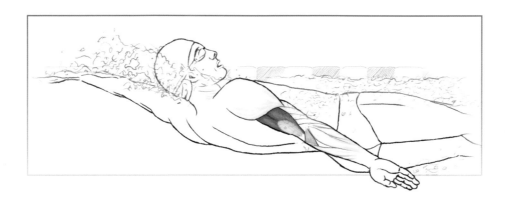

⚠️ **SAFETY TIP** As in swimming, your head must stay in alignment with your spine. Lifting your head up will lead to arching of the back, and looking down at your feet will roll your shoulders forward. Either action will take the spine out of its safe zone and increase the potential for an exercise-related injury.

VARIATION

Dumbbell Kickback With Tubing

This variation is useful when performing dryland exercises on a pool deck where no exercise bench is available to brace yourself. The amount of tension initially placed on the exercise cord should be light enough to allow you to reach the fully extended ending position. This exercise can be modified so that both arms do the kickbacks at the same time. Be sure to move in a slow, controlled manner and to avoid bouncing the upper body.

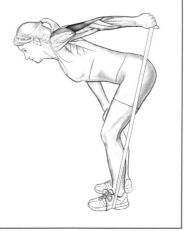

Close-Grip Push-Up

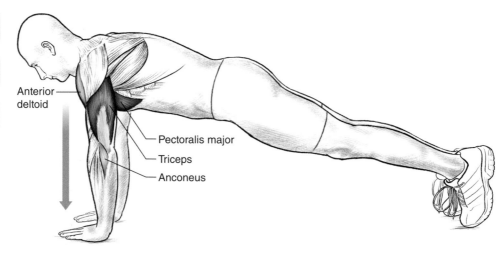

Anterior deltoid

Pectoralis major

Triceps

Anconeus

Execution

1. Facedown, slide both hands under your chest so that your thumbs touch along the midline of your body at nipple level. Your toes support your lower body.

2. Holding your body in a straight line from your ankles to the top of your head, push your upper body upward until the elbows are almost locked.

3. Lower your body until your chest is 1 inch (2.5 cm) off the ground.

Muscles Involved

Primary: Triceps brachii, pectoralis major

Secondary: Pectoralis minor, anterior deltoid, anconeus, wrist and finger flexors

⚠ **SAFETY TIP** If you are currently having shoulder pain or have a history of shoulder problems, avoid dropping too far into the ending position because doing so places extra stress on the shoulder joint. A good guideline to follow is to stop when the shoulders reach neutral. Because of the potential for increased stress on the shoulders, young swimmers who are still working to develop their overall shoulder strength should avoid this exercise.

Swimming Focus

Push-ups are one of the best dryland exercises because they can be performed anywhere and do not require any equipment. Another benefit is that they place the shoulder in what is called a closed-chain position; exercises that do this significantly enhance the recruitment of stabilizing muscles surrounding the shoulder joint.

While performing this or any other type of push-up, one of the main focuses should be on maintaining the body in a straight line from the ankles to the top of the head, just as if you were in a streamlined position in the water. A common mistake is to take the head out of line with the rest of the spine, which will lead to either arching of the back or dropping the hips to the ground. Maintaining proper form, especially a straight spine, is important; therefore, those who cannot maintain this position should modify the exercise by starting on their knees instead of their toes.

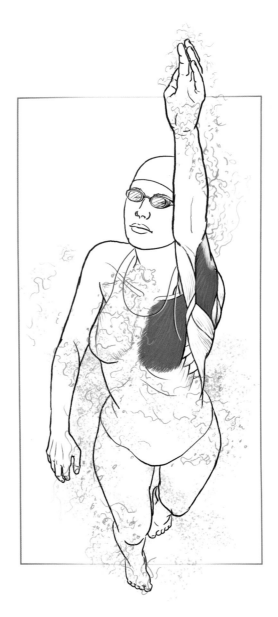

Close-Grip Push-Up With Medicine Ball

To increase the complexity and difficulty of this exercise, try using a medicine ball as the base of support. Choose a medicine ball that is approximately half the width of your chest. Position the ball so that its center is aligned with the middle of your chest and in line with your nipples.

Close-Grip Bench Press

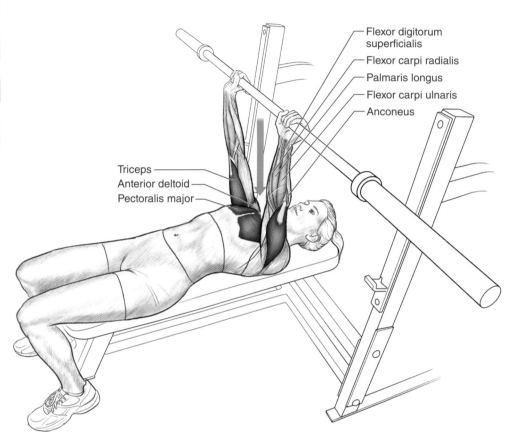

Flexor digitorum superficialis

Flexor carpi radialis

Palmaris longus

Flexor carpi ulnaris

Anconeus

Triceps

Anterior deltoid

Pectoralis major

Execution

1. Lie face up on a bench and grasp the bar using an overhand grip with your hands spaced 8 to 12 inches (20 to 30 cm) apart.
2. Lower the bar to a point just below the nipple line and allow your elbows to drift out at a 45-degree angle.
3. As soon as the bar touches your chest, reverse the movement.

Muscles Involved

Primary: Triceps brachii, pectoralis major

Secondary: Pectoralis minor, anterior deltoid, anconeus, wrist and finger flexors

Swimming Focus

This exercise has an advantage over close-grip push-ups because using weights as the form of resistance allows variation in the amount of stress placed on the triceps. Therefore, it can be used by swimmers who are unable to perform close-grip push-ups with the proper technique because of a lack of strength, as well as by swimmers who cannot sufficiently overload their triceps with close-grip push-ups because their triceps are so well developed.

When performing the exercise, allow the elbows to drift outward at a 45-degree angle to help isolate the triceps.

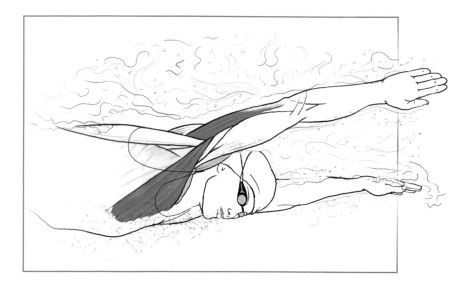

⚠️ **SAFETY TIP** From an injury prevention standpoint, the wrists must be kept in a neutral position when performing this exercise. If wrist pain occurs, try to increase the width of the grip. The exercise will target the triceps as long as the hand grip is less than shoulder-width. As an additional cautionary note, if you are currently experiencing shoulder pain or have a history of shoulder injury, modify how far you lower the bar by not letting the elbows pass below the level of the bench.

Before adding this exercise to a program, you should be comfortable with performing a normal bench press exercise as described in chapter 4 (page 70).

Tate Press

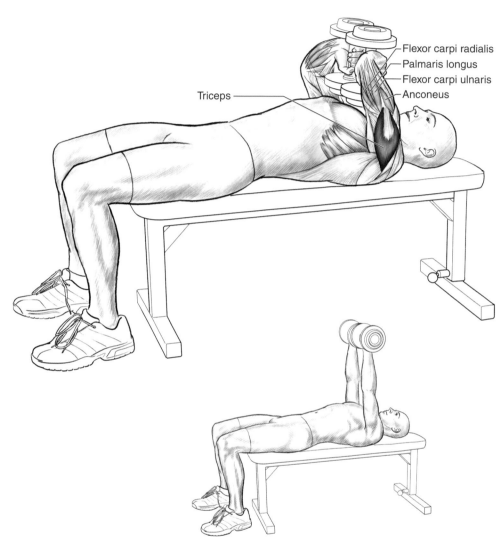

Flexor carpi radialis
Palmaris longus
Flexor carpi ulnaris
Anconeus
Triceps

Finish position.

Execution

1. Lying flat on a bench, gently rest two dumbbells on your chest so that your palms are facing your feet and your elbows are pointing straight out from your chest.

2. While maintaining the upper-arm and elbow position, begin to straighten your arms, keeping the dumbbells in contact with each other.

3. At the halfway point, begin to rotate the dumbbells from their starting vertical orientation to a horizontal orientation. Maintain the contact between the dumbbells for the entire time.

4. Continue pushing the dumbbells upward until your elbows are fully extended.

Muscles Involved

Primary: Triceps brachii

Secondary: Anconeus, wrist and finger flexors

Swimming Focus

The Tate press focuses on the lateral heads of the triceps brachii, making it a valuable exercise to include in a swimming dryland program.

One of the key components of this exercise is keeping the dumbbells in contact with each other during the entire exercise. To avoid potential injury, you must use an appropriate weight and avoid letting the dumbbells bounce off your chest when returning them to the starting position.

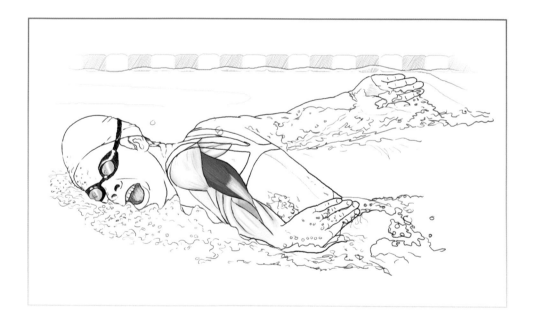

Barbell Biceps Curl

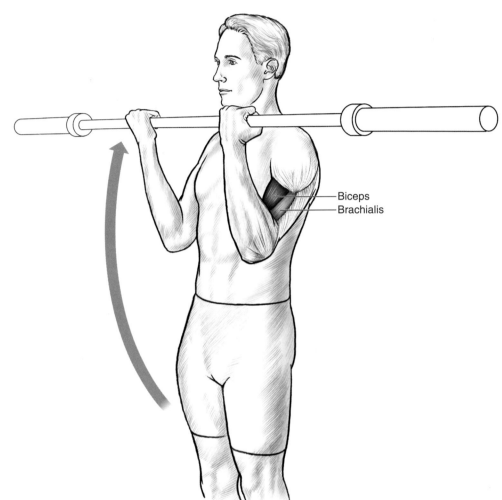

Biceps
Brachialis

Execution

1. Grasp the bar using an underhand grip. Your hands should be spaced shoulder-width apart.
2. Without leaning back, curl the bar toward your chest in an arc until the bar is level with your shoulders.
3. Return the bar to its start position at arm's length.

Muscles Involved

Primary: Biceps brachii

Secondary: Brachialis, forearm and finger flexors

Swimming Focus

Strengthening the biceps brachii and brachialis with this exercise will help with the initial catch component of the pull phase for backstroke. This exercise also enhances the second half of the pull phase during breaststroke. During these portions of the various strokes, maintaining the elbow in a flexed position is important. Loss of the flexed position by dropping the elbow during the freestyle catch, for example, leads to dramatic losses in power. The movements performed during this exercise also target the biceps brachii and brachialis in the same manner as they are utilized when performing flip turns.

An easy way to cheat when performing this exercise is to initiate a rocking motion with the upper body to generate extra momentum. You can minimize this tendency by performing the exercise with your back flat against a wall or by having a partner monitor your position.

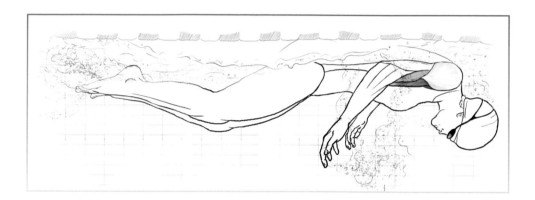

Dumbbell Biceps Curl

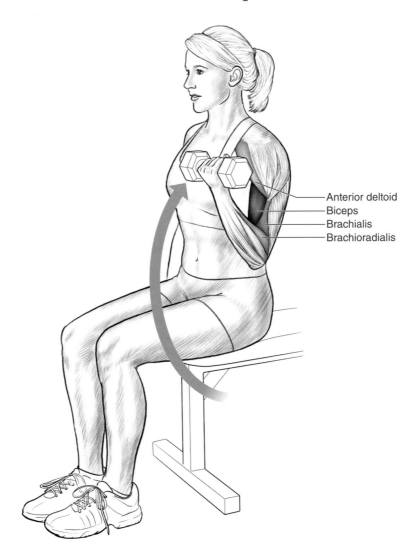

Anterior deltoid
Biceps
Brachialis
Brachioradialis

Execution

1. Sit at the end of a bench. With your arms fully extended, grasp a dumbbell in each hand with your palms facing inward.

2. One arm at a time, curl the dumbbell to your chest in an arc while at the same time slowly rotating your palm so that it faces your chest.

3. Alternate arms for each repetition.

Muscles Involved

Primary: Biceps brachii

Secondary: Anterior deltoid, brachialis, brachioradialis, supinator, forearm and finger flexors

Swimming Focus

The rotation of the palm inward (supination of the forearm) at the ending position places extra emphasis on the biceps brachii and mimics the final portion of the pull phase during breaststroke as you bring your palms in to the midline of your body.

Because it isolates one arm from the other, the dumbbell biceps curl overcomes a disadvantage of the barbell biceps curl. This exercise can be performed standing or sitting, but because of the alternating arm movements you should perform it seated to help maintain the upper torso in a fixed position.

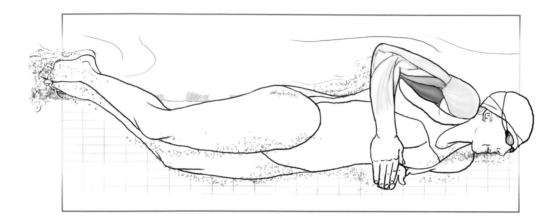

VARIATION

Biceps Curl With Tubing

An exercise cord allows you to incorporate this exercise into a poolside dryland program. The initial tension placed on the cord should be light enough to allow you to complete the entire range of motion.

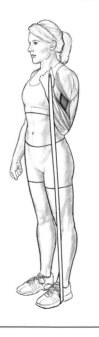

Concentration Curl

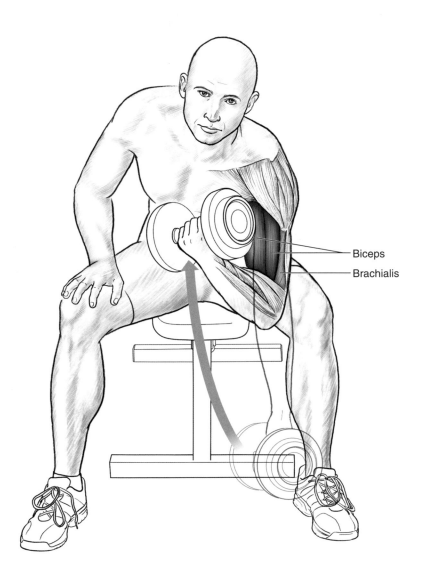

Biceps

Brachialis

Execution

1. Seated at the end of a bench, separate your legs so that they form a V and lean forward slightly with your torso.
2. While holding a dumbbell and bracing your elbow against the middle of your thigh, curl the dumbbell in an arc toward your shoulder.
3. Slowly lower the dumbbell back to the starting position.

Muscles Involved

Primary: Biceps brachii

Secondary: Brachialis, forearm and finger flexors

Swimming Focus

This exercise is useful if you are having difficulty maintaining your form with the barbell or dumbbell biceps curls or if you want to isolate the biceps brachii and brachialis. As the name implies, the primary purpose of this exercise is to concentrate on the curling motion and, in turn, to strengthen the elbow flexors. The key is to maintain the elbow in a stabilized position against the inner thigh and perform the exercise in a slow, controlled manner.

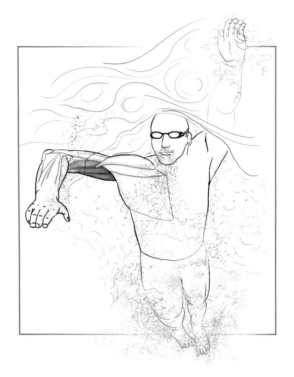

The shoulder girdle is important because it serves as the link between the arms and the trunk. It is the main rotation point about which all the arm movements take place during each of the four strokes. The shoulder girdle is composed of three bones: the clavicle (collarbone), scapula (shoulder blade), and humerus. Three joints make up the shoulder girdle: the sternoclavicular joint, which is the junction between the sternum (breastbone) and clavicle; the acromioclavicular joint, which is made up of the scapula and clavicle; and the glenohumeral joint, which is composed of the humerus and scapula. This chapter focuses on the movements that take place at the glenohumeral joint, which in layman's terms is the shoulder joint, and the movements of the scapula. The shoulder joint is one of the most flexible joints in the human body, as demonstrated by our ability to place our hands anywhere in our field of vision. This wide range of motion is possible because of the combination of six movements that occur at the shoulder girdle. Flexion involves raising the arm forward away from the body, as if you were raising your hand to answer a question. Extension, the reverse motion, involves lowering the hand from a flexed position. Moving your hand away from your body by raising it to the side is called abduction, and bringing your hand back toward the midline of your body is called adduction. The final two movements are rotational. External rotation involves rotation of the hand from the midline of the body in an outward motion. Internal rotation entails rotating your hand inward, as if you were bringing it in to rub your belly.

The muscles about the shoulder girdle can be classified into four groups: scapular pivoters, shoulder protectors, humeral positioners, and humeral propellers; an easy way to remember the four groups is to keep in mind the four Ps. The scapular pivoters are the trapezius, rhomboid major, rhomboid minor, serratus anterior, and pectoralis minor. As the name implies, these muscles are responsible for the upward and downward pivoting motion of the shoulder blade. They also account for the shoulder blade movements of elevation and depression and the movements of retraction and protraction. Upward rotation of the scapula is easily visualized if you stand behind a swimmer and watch him or her raise the arms to the sides up over the head. Elevation is simply the movement that occurs when you shrug your shoulders. Retraction is the movement performed when you pinch the shoulder blades together. A combination of these movements in unison with movement at the shoulder joint allows the wide variety of overhead movements that we are capable of performing. To observe the importance of these combined movements, place a hand on another person's shoulder blade. While you hold it in place, ask the person to lift a hand overhead. Notice the varied movements of the shoulder blade as the arm is moved through a variety of positions.

The trapezius is a large triangular muscle that attaches along the midline of the body to numerous points along the spine, starting at the base of the skull and ending at the bottom of the rib cage. From its attachment, the trapezius tapers outward to insert onto points on the clavicle and scapula. The trapezius can be divided into upper, middle, and lower portions. The upward portion is responsible for elevating and upwardly rotating the scapula. The middle portion aids in retraction, and the lower portion contributes to depression and downward rotation. The rhomboid major and minor run from the inner border of the shoulder blade

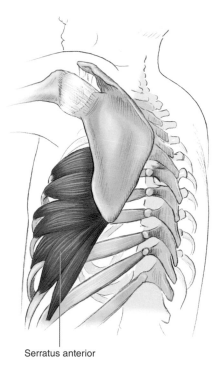

Serratus anterior

Figure 3.1   Serratus anterior.

to attachments on the spine. They work in conjunction with the middle portion of the trapezius to pinch the shoulder blades back. The serratus anterior is also attached along the inner border of the shoulder blade, but instead of running toward the midline, it runs in between the shoulder blade and the rib cage to attach along the outer surface of the first nine ribs (figure 3.1). Its two primary responsibilities are to assist in upward rotation of the scapula and to hold the scapula flat against the rib cage. Finally, the pectoralis minor is a small muscle on the front part of the rib cage that goes from an attachment on ribs 2 through 3 to a landmark on the superior aspect of the shoulder blade called the coracoid process. The pectoralis minor aids the lower fibers of the trapezius in depressing the scapula.

The scapular pivoters have three main areas of influence on the swimming athlete. First, proper upward rotation of the scapula is vital to allowing the swimmer to reach far out in front of the body when entering the hand into the water. The more elongated the swimmer can be, the more efficient the stroke will become. The second role is best described using the analogy that the shoulder blade and the scapular pivoters are like the foundation of a house. Building a spectacular house is foolish if the foundation is eventually going to crumble and fall apart. The same goes for the shoulder girdle and the scapula. If the scapular pivoters are weak, the rest of the kinetic chain making up the arms will eventually deteriorate and the risk of injury will increase. As discussed in chapter 2, when performing upper-extremity exercises, particularly those that target the shoulder joints, you should set the shoulder blades into a stable position. See the sidebar on page 13 for an explanation of how to set the shoulder blades. Lastly, strengthening the posterior scapular pivoters (trapezius, rhomboids, and serratus anterior) helps to overcome the forward rounded-shoulder posture commonly seen in swimmers because of overdevelopment of the latissimus dorsi.

The shoulder protector group, also known as the rotator cuff, is made up of the supraspinatus, infraspinatus, teres minor, and subscapularis (figure 3.2). The supraspinatus lies along the top part of the shoulder blade and attaches to the head of the humerus. The primary role of the supraspinatus is to help initiate overhead movements of the arm. The infraspinatus and teres minor arise from the back part of the scapula and attach next to the supraspinatus on the head of the humerus. The infraspinatus and teres minor act to rotate the shoulder externally. The subscapularis muscle runs along the front part of the shoulder, and like the other rotator cuff muscles, it originates on the scapula and inserts onto the head of the humerus. As the name implies, the primary action of the rotator cuff muscle group is to perform rotational movements at the shoulder joint. Because of the smaller sizes of these muscles, their contribution to the propulsive forces generated while swimming are relatively small; they do, however, have an important role in aiding in the recovery phase of all the strokes. Another vitally important role is their "cuff" function, which stabilizes the shoulder joint. When considering the role of the rotator cuff in stabilizing the shoulder joint, remember that the shoulder is a ball-and-socket joint that resembles a golf ball sitting on a tee. The rotator cuff muscles act as dynamic stabilizers by creating opposing forces that keep the ball centered on the tee. In some instances an imbalance can arise amongst the

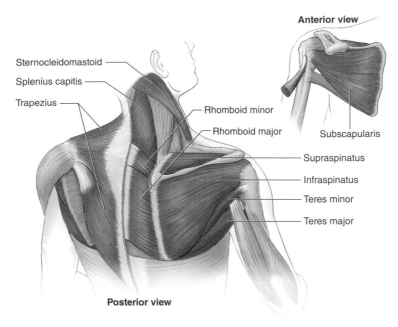

Sternocleidomastoid

Splenius capitis

Trapezius

Rhomboid minor

Rhomboid major

Anterior view

Subscapularis

Supraspinatus

Infraspinatus

Teres minor

Teres major

Posterior view

Figure 3.2 Shoulder blade and neck.

rotator cuff muscles, which inhibits their stabilizing mechanism and in turn increases the risk of injury. The shoulder joint sacrifices stability in favor of mobility and therefore depends on the rotator cuff muscle group to act as stabilizers and protectors.

The next major muscle group is the positioner group, which is actually only one muscle that has three separate divisions—anterior, middle, and posterior. The deltoid is the shoulder cap muscle that drapes over the upper portion of the shoulder joint (figure 3.3). The deltoid is called the positioner group because it is the primary muscle involved in changing the position of the humerus and thus the entire arm. The anterior portion is responsible for flexing and internally rotating the shoulder joint. The posterior portion performs the opposite movements, extension and external rotation. The middle portion is responsible for lifting the arm to the side, which is the movement of abduction. The deltoid is most active during the recovery phase. Each portion plays an important role in moving the arm during the various stages of the recovery phase.

The final muscle group, the propellers, includes the latissimus dorsi and pectoralis major. This name is derived from the fact that these muscles are the primary force generators at the shoulder joint. Because of the large number of exercises that target these muscles, their contributions to the movement of a swimmer and associated exercises will be reviewed in the chapters covering the chest and back.

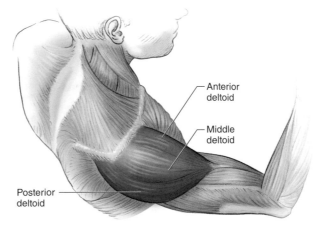

Anterior deltoid

Middle deltoid

Posterior deltoid

Figure 3.3 Deltoid.

Forward Dumbbell Deltoid Raise

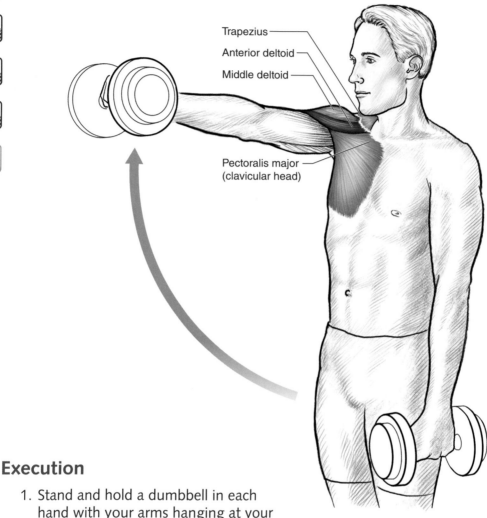

Trapezius
Anterior deltoid
Middle deltoid
Pectoralis major (clavicular head)

Execution

1. Stand and hold a dumbbell in each hand with your arms hanging at your sides and your palms facing your thighs.
2. Holding a slight bend in your elbows, raise the right dumbbell forward until it is level with your shoulders.
3. As you raise the dumbbell, slowly rotate your hands so that your palm faces the floor at the end of the exercise.
4. As you begin lowering the right dumbbell, initiate the movement of the left dumbbell.

Muscles Involved

Primary: Anterior deltoid

Secondary: Middle deltoid, trapezius, pectoralis major (clavicular head)

Swimming Focus

The anterior deltoid, the primary muscle engaged throughout this exercise, is a key player in the recovery process of butterfly, breaststroke, and especially backstroke. During butterfly it is active during the second half of the recovery, and during breaststroke it contributes by guiding the movements of the arm and hand from underneath the swimmer's chest to a fully extended and elongated position, maximizing the efficiency of the stroke. The entire recovery phase of backstroke, from water exit until reentry, also relies on recruitment of the anterior deltoid. As the speed of the stroke increases and the need for rapid recovery increases, so does the demand placed on the muscle.

You can use this exercise to build on the scapular setting motion previously described. To do this exercise, stand with a tall, upright posture and focus on pinching your shoulder blade backward and downward. While holding it in this set position, perform the exercise. Have a partner monitor your movements from behind to make sure that you do not start to shrug your shoulders.

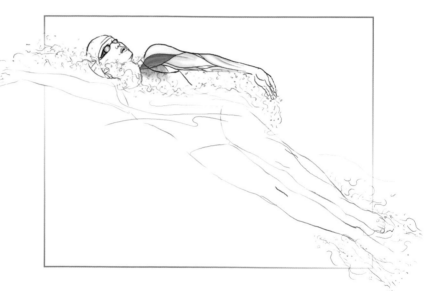

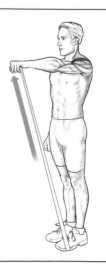

VARIATION

Forward Deltoid Raise With Tubing

Tubing targets the same muscles, but because of the ease of varying the resistance by simply stretching or slackening the exercise tubing, this variation may be better than the dumbbell variation for an on-deck dryland program.

Lateral Dumbbell Deltoid Raise

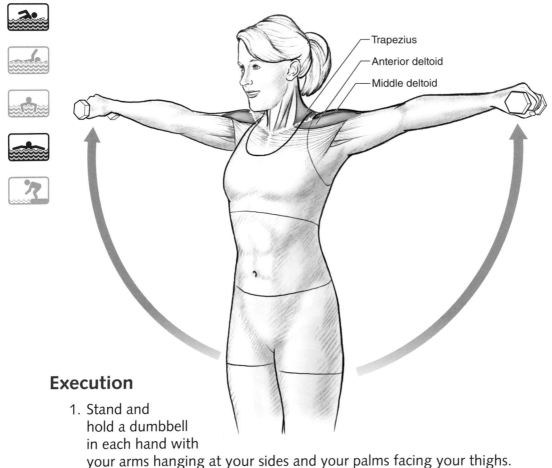

Trapezius
Anterior deltoid
Middle deltoid

Execution

1. Stand and hold a dumbbell in each hand with your arms hanging at your sides and your palms facing your thighs.
2. With a slight bend in your elbows, raise the dumbbells to the side until they are level with your shoulders.
3. Slowly lower the dumbbells.

Muscles Involved

Primary: Middle deltoid

Secondary: Anterior deltoid, posterior deltoid, supraspinatus, trapezius

Swimming Focus

The primary focus of this exercise is the middle deltoid, one of the key muscles involved in the recovery phase of freestyle and butterfly. Unlike freestyle, butterfly lacks a body roll to aid in arm recovery, leading to heavy reliance on the deltoid muscle group, particularly the middle deltoid, to reposition the arm. As with the forward dumbbell deltoid raise, you should emphasize a tall, upright posture when performing this exercise. Like the forward dumbbell deltoid raise, this exercise is a good fundamental starting point for you to practice setting your scapula when performing upper-extremity exercises.

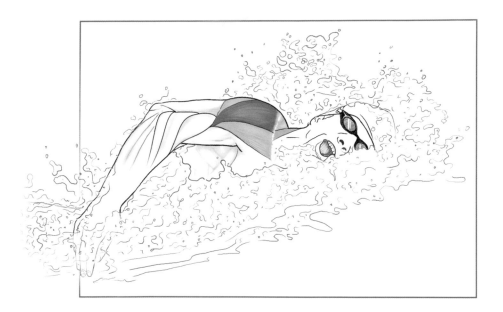

⚠ **SAFETY TIP** To avoid overstressing the rotator cuff muscles, which are stabilizing the shoulder joint during the exercise, do not raise the dumbbells above shoulder height.

VARIATIONS

Lateral Deltoid Raise With Tubing

Tubing targets the same muscles, but because of the ease of varying the resistance by simply stretching or slackening the exercise tubing, this variation may be better than the dumbbell variation for an on-deck dryland program.

Overhead C

As mentioned previously, raising the arms above the level of the shoulders while the palms are facing down can be detrimental. The addition of the C at the end range changes the position of the shoulders in a way that allows movement of the arms above shoulder height while alleviating the concern of causing excessive stress to the rotator cuff. To complete the C movement, envision each hand as the hand of a clock. Starting in the 6 o'clock position with your palms facing down, rotate both upward in a clockwise manner to the 12 o'clock position.

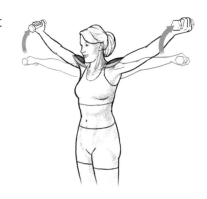

T Exercise

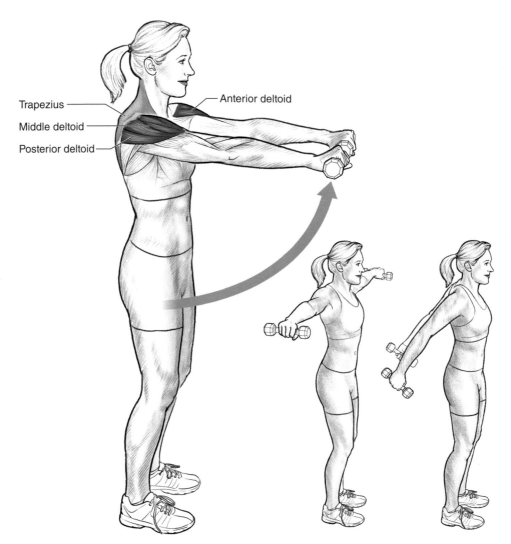

Trapezius

Anterior deltoid

Middle deltoid

Posterior deltoid

Forward raise.　　　**Lateral raise.**　　　**Backward raise.**

Execution

1. With a dumbbell in each hand, raise your hands forward until the dumbbells are level with your shoulders.

2. Return to the starting position and then raise the dumbbells laterally, again until they are level with your shoulders.

3. Return to the starting position and then lift the dumbbells back behind your torso at approximately 45 degrees.

4. Start again with the forward raise.

Muscles Involved

Primary: Anterior deltoid, middle deltoid, posterior deltoid

Secondary: Supraspinatus, trapezius

Swimming Focus

This exercise targets all three portions of the deltoid (anterior, middle, and posterior), making it an excellent all-around exercise for strengthening the shoulders. As a result, it strengthens the recovery phase of all four strokes. For the younger swimmer first entering the sport, this is a good exercise for the initial development of shoulder strength, which will be important as the swimmer progresses and increases yardage gradually. For the older swimmer, because of the multiple movements targeted, this exercise is better suited for building endurance at the beginning of the season or when recovering from an injury.

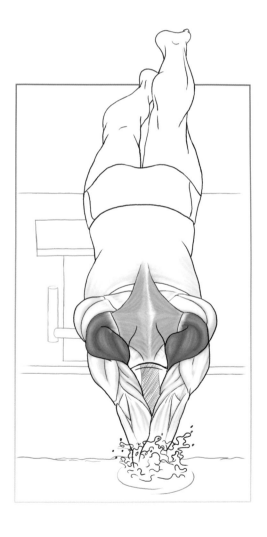

Dumbbell Shoulder Press

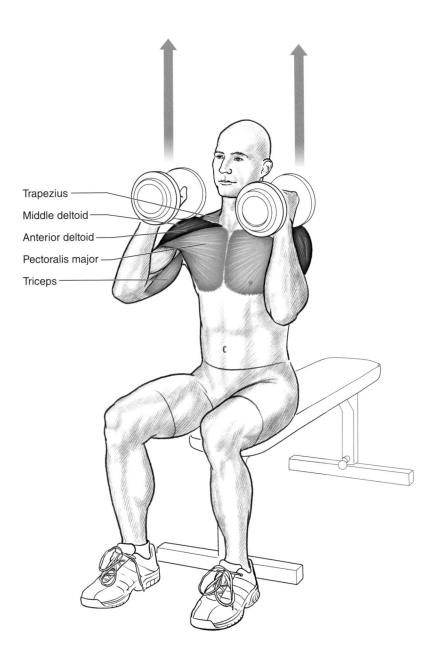

Trapezius
Middle deltoid
Anterior deltoid
Pectoralis major
Triceps

Execution

1. Sitting up straight, hold the dumbbells at shoulder level with your elbows in and your palms facing your body.
2. Press the dumbbells upward until your elbows are almost locked.
3. Slowly lower to the starting position.

Muscles Involved

Primary: Anterior deltoid, middle deltoid

Secondary: Pectoralis major, posterior deltoid, trapezius, supraspinatus, triceps brachii

Swimming Focus

To maximize the distanced gained during each stroke, you need to be able to enter the water with your arm or arms extended and your body in an elongated position. This exercise helps develop overhead strength and confidence in extending your reach when entering the water.

The exercise described here is a modified version of the military press motion performed in traditional weight lifting. The traditional version is usually performed with the dumbbells held in the "stick 'em up" position, with the palms rotated outward. Swimmer should avoid this position because it can place undue stress on the shoulders and could be detrimental when combined with the stress already present from the yardage load in the water.

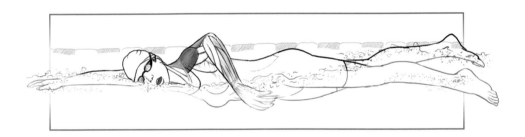

⚠ **SAFETY TIP** Because of the overhead nature of the exercise, young swimmers who may not have the strength and coordination to control the movement should not perform it. If you are currently experiencing shoulder pain or have a recent history of it, you should follow the 90/90 rule when performing this and other upper-extremity exercises. The 90/90 rule states that you should avoid dropping your shoulder below 90 degrees of abduction or flexion and avoid flexing your elbow more than 90 degrees.

Bent-Over Reverse Dumbbell Fly

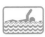

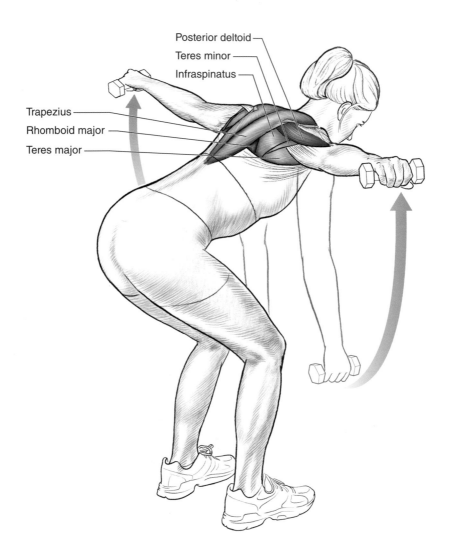

Posterior deltoid

Teres minor

Infraspinatus

Trapezius

Rhomboid major

Teres major

Execution

1. Standing with a flat back, bend forward at your waist until your back is near parallel to the ground.

2. With your arms hanging, hold the dumbbells so that your palms face in.

3. Keeping your arms straight, raise the dumbbells in an arcing motion until your elbows are level with your shoulders.

4. Resisting gravity, slowly return to the starting position.

Muscles Involved

Primary: Rhomboid major, rhomboid minor, posterior deltoid

Secondary: Trapezius, infraspinatus, teres major, teres minor

Swimming Focus

This exercise can have two points of emphasis depending on the weight of the dumbbell used. Using lighter weights allows you to concentrate more on pinching the shoulder blades together at the end of the exercise, thus focusing on recruiting the rhomboid major and rhomboid minor. This is an effective way to target the rhomboids to improve their role as a dynamic stabilizer of the shoulder blades, which in turn will increase the foundational strength of the shoulder blades and decrease the risk of injury. As the weight increases, the emphasis shifts from the rhomboids to the posterior deltoid along the back of the shoulder. Targeting either of these muscle groups with this exercise will transfer to strengthening the recovery phase of breaststroke and butterfly, as well as contribute to the initial portion of the recovery during freestyle.

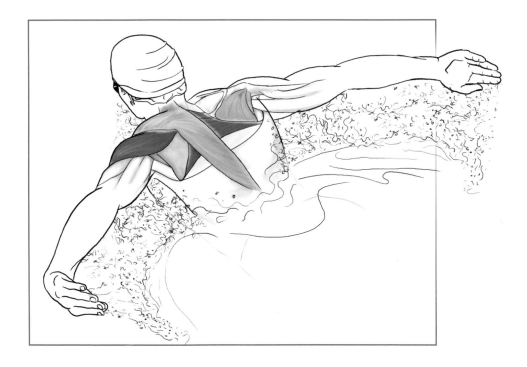

⚠ **SAFETY TIP** Be sure to keep your head in line with your back when performing this exercise. Lifting your head will lead to arching of the low back, and dropping your head will cause rounding of the upper back. Either motion can place unnecessary stress on the low to mid-back.

Prone T, Y, A (Blackburn)

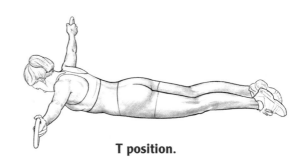

T position.

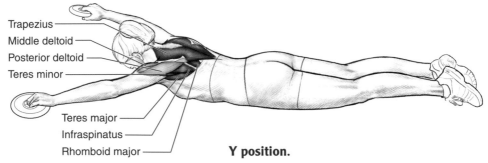

Trapezius
Middle deltoid
Posterior deltoid
Teres minor

Teres major
Infraspinatus
Rhomboid major

Y position.

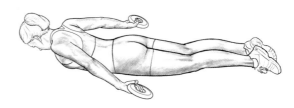

A position.

Execution

1. Lying facedown, slightly arch your upper back and lift your shoulders off the ground.
2. In a T position with your thumbs pointing to the ceiling, oscillate your hands up and down for 30 seconds.
3. Switching to the Y position with your palms down, oscillate your hands up and down for 30 seconds.
4. Finish with your hands down by your sides forming an A. With your palms up, oscillate your hands up and down for 30 seconds.

Muscles Involved

Primary: Rhomboid major, rhomboid minor, infraspinatus, teres major, teres minor, supraspinatus, trapezius

Secondary: Anterior deltoid, middle deltoid, posterior deltoid

Swimming Focus

Because of the variety of shoulder positions used, this exercise targets most of the muscles that support the shoulder blade (scapular stabilizers). Performing this exercise will help to enhance the stability of the shoulder blade, which will aid in transferring the forces generated by the arms to the rest of the body while swimming and help prevent shoulder injuries.

During the exercise the focus is on squeezing the shoulder blades together and performing small, rapid oscillatory movements with the arms. As endurance improves and you are able to maintain good form while holding each of the three positions for 60 seconds, you can incorporate weights as shown to make the exercise more challenging. These muscles are small, so any weights used should be very light (1.25 to 2.5 lb, or .55 to 1.1 kg, to start) and changes should be made in small increments.

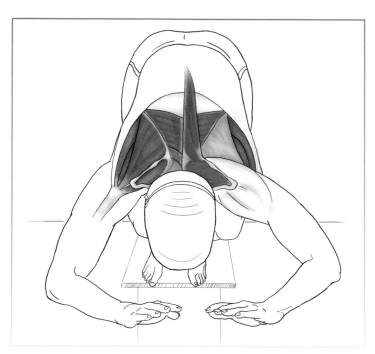

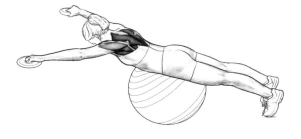

VARIATION

Physioball T, Y, A

Although adding a physioball makes the exercise much more challenging, it more closely mimics the demands encountered while swimming. As in the water, holding the body in a straight line from the feet all the way to the top of the head is important.

Scapular Push-Up

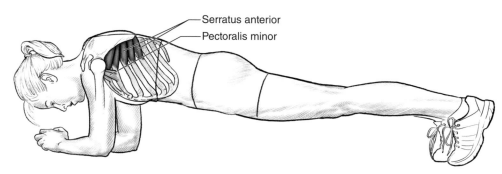

Serratus anterior
Pectoralis minor

Execution

1. Facedown, support your body weight on your toes and forearms.
2. Holding your body in a straight line, lower your chest while maintaining the shoulder position and allowing your shoulder blades to pinch together.
3. By rolling your shoulders (protraction), push your upper body upward.

Muscles Involved

Primary: Serratus anterior

Secondary: Pectoralis minor

Swimming Focus

The sole target of this exercise is a muscle called the serratus anterior, which is important in keeping your shoulder blade tight against your back. Weakness of this muscle will lead to "winging" of the shoulder blade, a sign that the shoulder blade is not being properly controlled, which in turn increases the risk of shoulder injury. The serratus anterior is also important in rotating the shoulder blade upward when moving overhead, which helps to extend the stroke.

The purpose of performing this exercise from the forearms instead of the hands is to isolate the movements to the shoulder region.

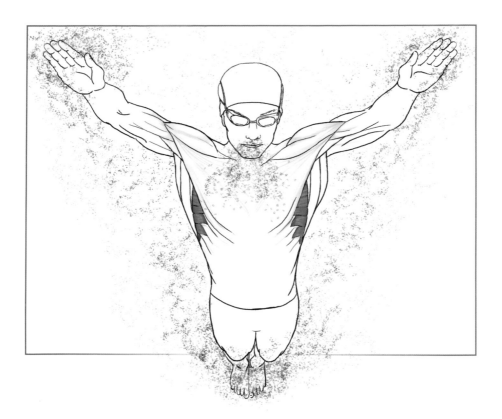

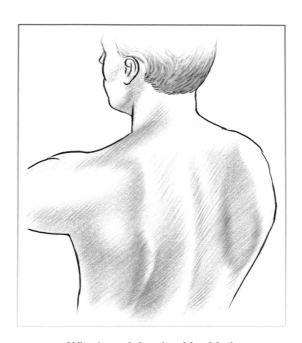

Winging of the shoulder blade.

Scapular Dip

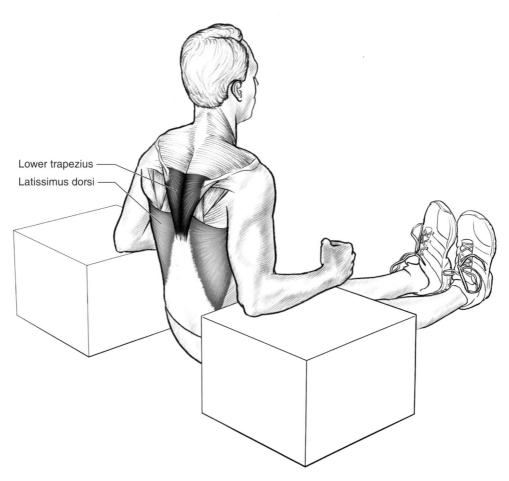

Lower trapezius

Latissimus dorsi

Execution

1. Sitting upright between two 6-inch (15 cm) boxes, position your hands so that they are in line with your torso. Your elbows should be flexed to 90 degrees, which will allow you to rest your forearms on the box.

2. Pushing down, lift your butt off the ground, emphasizing a reverse shrug of your shoulders.

3. Lower back down until you barely touch the ground and repeat.

Muscles Involved

Primary: Lower trapezius

Secondary: Pectoralis major, pectoralis minor, latissimus dorsi

Swimming Focus

This exercise helps to increase the stability of the shoulder joint and to correct postural changes frequently seen in swimmers. It targets the lower fibers of the trapezius, where weakness can lead to shoulder injuries. Strengthening of the lower fibers of the trapezius also helps to correct the forward rounded-shoulder posture common to swimmers.

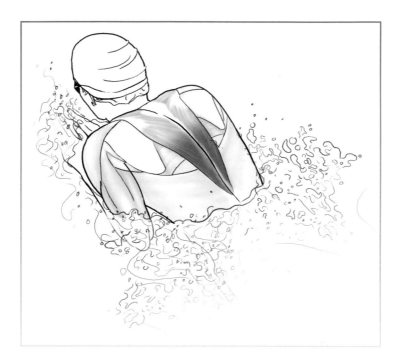

Internal Rotation With Tubing

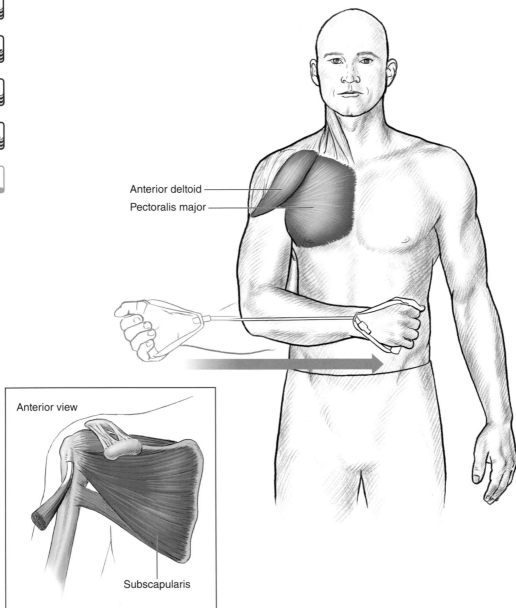

Anterior deltoid

Pectoralis major

Anterior view

Subscapularis

Execution

1. Stand sideways 4 feet (120 cm) from a pole with a piece of exercise tubing attached at elbow height. Hold the end of the tubing with the arm closer to it and bend the elbow to 90 degrees.

2. Rotate your hand across the front of your body until it contacts your torso. Keep your forearm parallel to the floor during the entire movement.

3. Slowly return to the starting position.

Muscles Involved

Primary: Subscapularis

Secondary: Pectoralis major, latissimus dorsi, anterior deltoid

Swimming Focus

The subscapularis is one of the four rotator cuff muscles, a muscle group that is important in stabilizing the shoulder joint during repetitive upper-extremity exercises; hence, exercises that target the subscapularis play a vital role in injury prevention. Remember that the rotator cuff muscles all arise from the shoulder blade, so when performing this exercise you should stabilize the shoulder blade by pinching it down and back and holding that position during the exercise. Placing a towel between your elbow and the side of your body as shown helps decrease tension on some key muscles and serves as a reminder to keep the elbow tight against your side as you rotate your arm.

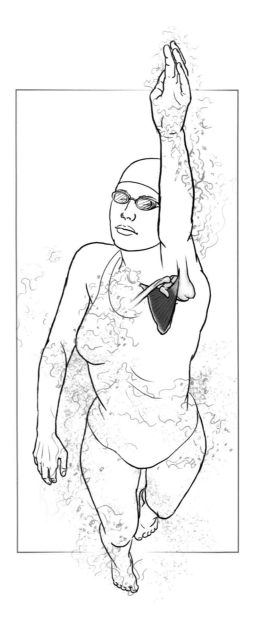

External Rotation With Tubing

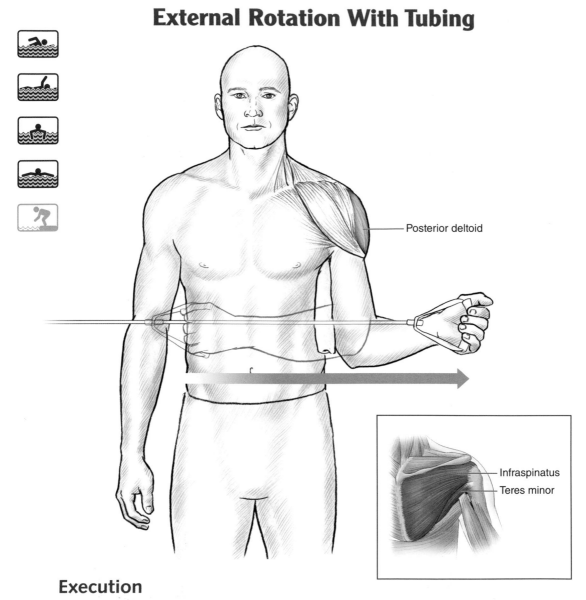

Posterior deltoid

Infraspinatus
Teres minor

Execution

1. Stand sideways 4 feet (120 cm) from a pole with a piece of exercise tubing attached at elbow height. Hold the tubing in the hand farther from the pole and bend the elbow to 90 degrees.

2. Rotate your hand away from your torso until you have covered a 90-degree arc. Keep your forearm parallel to the floor during the entire movement.

3. Slowly return to the starting position.

Muscles Involved

Primary: Infraspinatus, teres minor

Secondary: Posterior deltoid

Swimming Focus

External rotation isolates the infraspinatus and teres minor, two components of the rotator cuff muscle group. These muscles are important in stabilizing the shoulder joint during repetitive upper-extremity exercises. Because all the strokes except backstroke emphasize internal rotation movements at the shoulder, adding this exercise to address the strength imbalance is important.

Remember that the rotator cuff muscles all arise from the shoulder blade, so you must stabilize the shoulder blade when performing this exercise. Pinch your shoulder blade down and back and hold that position during the exercise. Placing a towel between your elbow and the side of your body as shown helps decrease tension on some key muscles and reminds you to keep your elbow tight against your side as you rotate your arm.

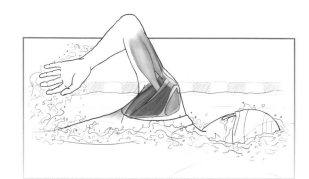

VARIATIONS

Side-Lying Dumbbell External Rotation

From a side-lying position, with your elbow bent to 90 degrees, rotate your arm so that the dumbbell moves away from your abdomen in an arcing motion toward the ceiling. Avoid twisting your upper body because doing so will take the isolation away from the shoulder joint. Dumbbells provide a more consistent form of resistance than the exercise tubing.

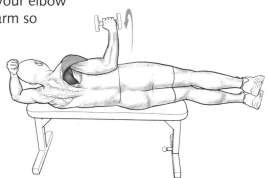

Double-Arm External Rotation

Perform this variation by holding both arms in the starting position for the external rotation with tubing exercise. Hold one end of an exercise tube in each hand. In this starting position, there should be a small amount of tension on the tubing. Next, rotate both arms outward 45 degrees while simultaneously pinching your shoulder blades together. Hold this position for three to four seconds and then return to the starting position.

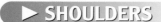

Crabwalk

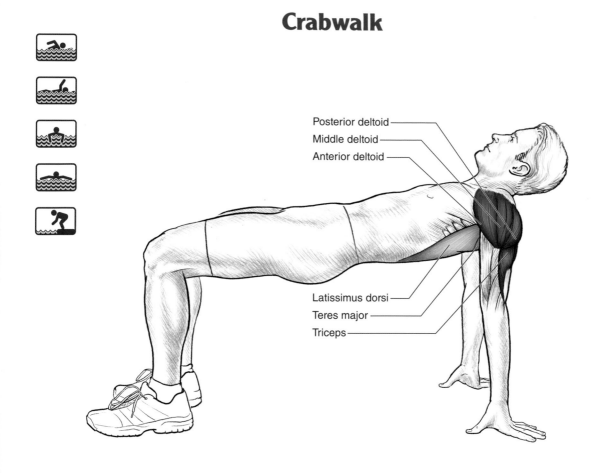

Posterior deltoid
Middle deltoid
Anterior deltoid

Latissimus dorsi
Teres major
Triceps

Execution

1. Position your hands and feet so that they are flat on the ground and you are face up.
2. Lift your butt up off the ground by tightening your gluteal muscles.
3. Begin "walking" by first moving your hands and then your feet.
4. Avoid excessive shoulder strain by moving your hands no more than 6 to 8 inches (15 to 20 cm) at a time.

Muscles Involved

Primary: Anterior deltoid, middle deltoid, posterior deltoid, rotator cuff (supraspinatus, infraspinatus, teres minor, subscapularis), triceps brachii

Secondary: Latissimus dorsi, teres major

Swimming Focus

This excellent all-around exercise targets the deltoids, rotator cuff, and triceps brachii, all of which contribute to each of the four competitive strokes. Recruitment of the deltoid will transfer to gains in the recovery phase of each stroke. Strengthening the rotator cuff will help develop shoulder stability, and the triceps brachii is a varying contributor to the propulsive phase of each stroke. Additionally, the reaching-back movement performed during the exercise will help develop better awareness of where the hand is in relation to the body, which will improve swimming mechanics.

Another benefit is that the exercise places the shoulder in a closed-chain position. Exercises that do this enhance the recruitment of stabilizing muscles surrounding the shoulder joint. The term *closed chain* means that the anchor point of the exercise, in this case the hand, is in contact with the ground.

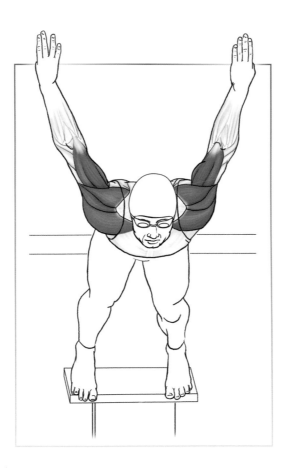

Overhead Single-Arm Bounce

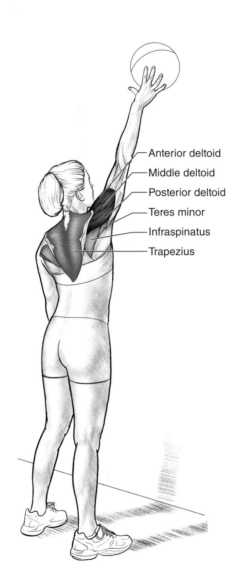

Anterior deltoid
Middle deltoid
Posterior deltoid
Teres minor
Infraspinatus
Trapezius

Execution

1. Position yourself so that you are standing 12 inches (30 cm) from a wall. Begin by holding an air-filled ball (for example, a soccer ball) in the palm of your hand, as a waiter would hold a serving tray overhead.

2. Initiate the bouncing motion by moving your entire arm. The target on the wall is either the 11 o'clock (left arm) position or 1 o'clock (right arm) position.

3. Emphasize small, rapid bounces.

Muscles Involved

Primary: Anterior deltoid, middle deltoid, posterior deltoid

Secondary: Trapezius, rotator cuff (supraspinatus, infraspinatus, teres minor, subscapularis)

Swimming Focus

This exercise is useful for developing strength when the hand is in an overhead position, which will increase your confidence when you are trying to elongate your stroke. The hand positioning with this exercise closely mimics that seen with freestyle and butterfly. As a result this exercise can be beneficial in developing a quick transition from the catch portion of both strokes to the pulling portion.

When performing the bouncing motion, emphasize small, rapid movements to focus on the deltoid and rotator cuff. This exercise builds endurance in the scapular stabilizing and rotator cuff muscles, which aids in the prevention of injuries. If you use larger movements, you recruit the pectoralis major and latissimus dorsi, which is not the goal of this exercise.

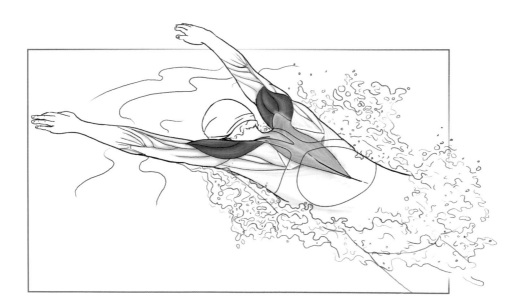

The primary muscle of the chest, the pectoralis major, is one of two humeral propeller muscles involved in generating most of the forces that propel a swimmer through the water. With the aid of the shoulder girdle muscles described in chapter 3 and the muscles of the arm described in chapter 2, the forces generated by the pectoralis major are transmitted to the hand and forearm, which serve as the primary force conduits through which a swimmer guides the body through the water. Other muscles in the chest region are the pectoralis minor and the serratus anterior.

The pectoralis major (figure 4.1 on page 62) is typically divided into two heads: the clavicular (upper) head and the sternal (lower) head. The clavicular portion comprises the upper portion of the pectoralis major and arises from the anterior surface of the inner half of the clavicle. The sternal portion forms the lower portion and arises from the anterior surface of the sternum and the cartilage of the first six ribs. The upper and lower portions join and cross the shoulder joint, attaching to the humerus. As the pectoralis major contracts and pulls on the humerus, the following movements take place at the shoulder joint: flexion, extension, adduction, and internal rotation. Flexion involves bringing the arm from the side of the body forward. Extension, the reverse of flexion, involves returning the arm to the side from a flexed position. Adduction involves bringing the arm toward the midline of the body when it has been raised to the side; this movement can be either horizontal or vertical in nature. Internal rotation involves rotating the hand across the body so that the palm is resting on the abdomen. For an in-depth description of the pectoralis minor and serratus anterior, refer to the introduction to chapter 3. For this chapter it is best to think of their role in helping to stabilize the shoulder blade and in turn the shoulder joint as the pectoralis major acts on the humerus. A number of other muscles are also activated during the exercises described in this chapter. The anterior deltoid often functions to assist the pectoralis major with shoulder flexion. The latissimus dorsi assists with shoulder extension, and the triceps brachii functions to extend the elbow joint during the many pressing exercises that target the pectoralis major.

As previously mentioned, the pectoralis major is one of two primary force generators acting to propel a swimmer through the water. During freestyle and butterfly, as the hand first enters into the water and the body is in an elongated position, the pectoralis major initiates the pulling phase of both strokes. At this time the upper portion of the pectoralis major is a key contributor to the movement. As the hand moves toward its anchor point, the lower portion along with the latissimus dorsi joins in to assist in propelling the swimmer through the water. As the hand passes below the shoulder joint, the contribution of the upper portion of the pectoralis major

Medicine Ball Push-Up

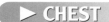

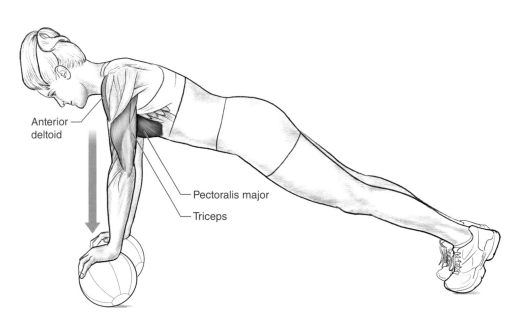

Anterior deltoid

Pectoralis major

Triceps

Execution

1. Position two medicine balls shoulder-width apart. Place one hand on each ball. Support your lower body on your toes.
2. Holding your body in a straight line from your ankles to the top of your head, push your upper body upward until your elbows are almost locked.
3. Lower your body until your chest is 1 inch (2.5 cm) off the ground.

Muscles Involved

Primary: Pectoralis major

Secondary: Anterior deltoid, triceps brachii

⚠ **SAFETY TIP** Lowering the chest too far can place extra stress on the anterior part of the shoulder. Those with a shoulder injury or a history of one should avoid this movement.

Swimming Focus

Incorporating medicine balls is an effective way to increase the difficulty of the push-up exercise for a person who can consistently maintain proper technique when performing regular push-ups.
The unstable nature of the medicine balls places increased demand on the shoulder and core-stabilizing musculature, which will have to react to the hands being anchored on an unstable surface. Additionally, the altered hand position allows a larger available range of motion when performing the exercise, which will strengthen the muscles through a larger range.

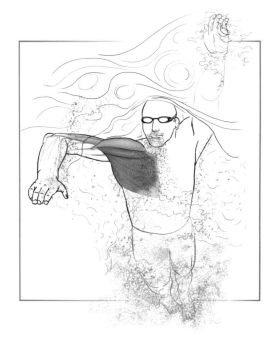

VARIATION

Medicine Ball Push-Up
With Staggered Hand Placement

The staggered hand placement (one hand on a medicine ball and one hand on the floor) creates a challenging scenario because each hand is in a different position. The challenge is similar to that encountered when swimming freestyle and backstroke. The altered hand position places more strengthening emphasis on the hand on the medicine ball. Additionally, the added rotation of the trunk alters the demands placed on the abdominal core musculature.

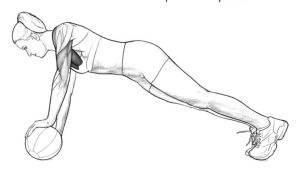

Barbell Flat Bench Press

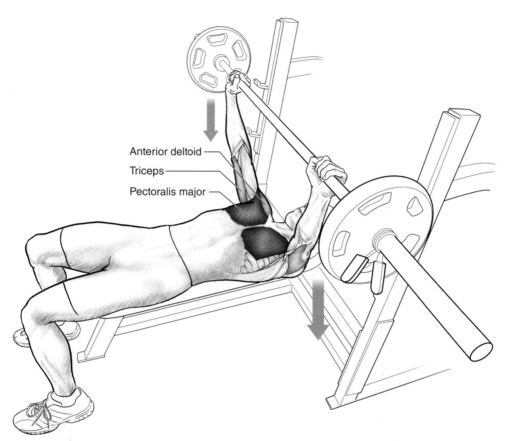

Anterior deltoid

Triceps

Pectoralis major

Execution

1. Lie flat on the bench and position your feet shoulder-width apart and flat on the floor.
2. Grasp the bar with an overhand grip with your arms straight and your hands approximately shoulder-width apart.
3. Slowly lower the bar until it just barely touches the middle of your chest.
4. Drive the bar upward until your elbows are extended.

Muscles Involved

Primary: Pectoralis major

Secondary: Anterior deltoid, triceps brachii

Swimming Focus

The bench press is the primary exercise used in almost all athletic realms to strengthen the pectoralis major. This exercise allows you to strengthen the pectoralis major through a wide range of motion, which will carry over to strengthening the pull phase of freestyle, butterfly, and breaststroke. Although it uses the same muscle groups as push-ups do, the resistance can be varied, overcoming one of the disadvantages of push-ups. Lowering the bar to the middle of the chest (nipple line) is important; doing this helps bring the elbows down along the side of the body. Lowering the bar to a point on the upper chest (like the clavicles) keeps the elbows high, placing undo stress on the anterior part of the shoulder.

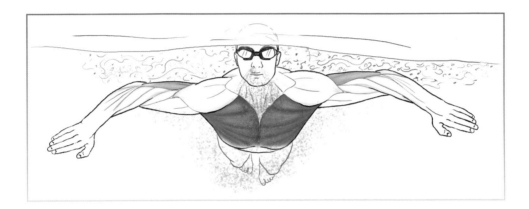

VARIATION

Dumbbell Flat Bench Press

Using dumbbells allows the hands to move independently of each other, creating an exercise that more closely relates to the independent demands encountered while swimming. Using dumbbells also allows the arms to be isolated from one another, which prevents a stronger arm from compensating for a weaker arm.

Dumbbell Physioball Bench Press

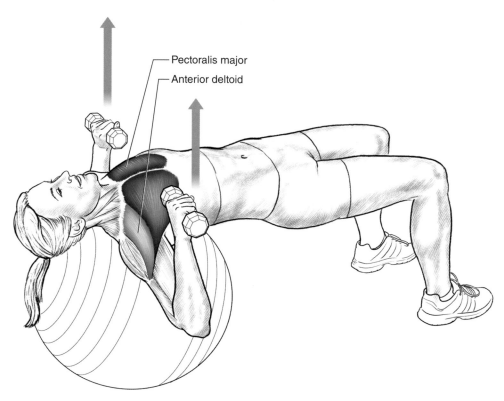

Pectoralis major

Anterior deltoid

Execution

1. Holding a dumbbell in each hand, sit on the physioball.
2. Slide down into a bridge position with your neck and shoulders balanced on the ball.
3. While keeping your hips straight, lower the dumbbells to the level of your chest.
4. Press the dumbbells upward until your elbows are almost locked.

Muscles Involved

Primary: Pectoralis major

Secondary: Anterior deltoid, triceps brachii

Swimming Focus

This exercise has the same benefits as the dumbbell variation of the barbell flat bench press but has the added benefit of requiring you to activate additional muscle groups to maintain body position. Having only the feet and shoulders as contact points supporting the body places high demands on the stabilizing muscles of both the torso and the hips. Because of the unstable nature of the physioball, the stabilizing muscles that are functioning to maintain body position are constantly being challenged.

While performing the exercise, the hips and torso should be held in a position in which a straight line can be drawn from the knees, through the hips and torso, to the top of the head. Maintaining this body position mimics the demands encountered while holding a streamlined position. As with other exercises, excessive arching or rounding of the low back increases the risk of injury.

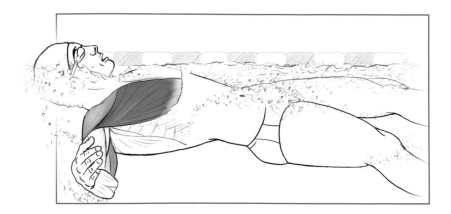

⚠️ **SAFETY TIP** Young swimmers should not perform this exercise until they have demonstrated proper bench-pressing technique on a stable bench.

Barbell Incline Bench Press

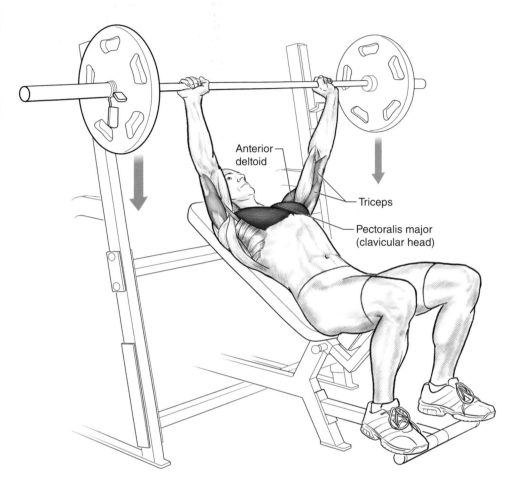

Anterior deltoid

Triceps

Pectoralis major (clavicular head)

Execution

1. Sit on an incline bench (angled between 45 and 60 degrees) and position your feet shoulder-width apart.
2. Grasp the bar with an overhand grip and place your hands about shoulder-width apart above your chest.
3. Slowly lower the bar until it just barely touches your upper chest.
4. Drive the bar upward until your elbows are fully extended.

Muscles Involved

Primary: Pectoralis major (clavicular head)

Secondary: Anterior deltoid, middle deltoid, triceps brachii

Swimming Focus

The elevated upper-body position places the focus of this exercise on the clavicular (upper) portion of the pectoralis major and the anterior and middle deltoids. The advantage of isolating the upper portion of the pectoralis major is that it is active during the initial portion of the pull phase during freestyle, butterfly, and breaststroke. Targeted strengthening of the muscle in this position will not only enhance the strength of the initial portion of the pull but also improve your confidence in elongating your stroke.

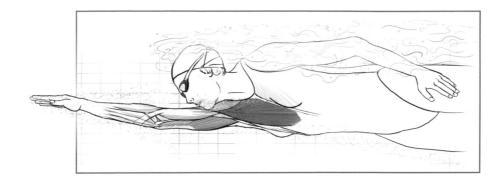

⚠ SAFETY TIP Keys to protecting the shoulder joint and avoiding injury include lowering the bar to a point at the middle of the chest (nipple line) and not allowing the hands and barbell to shift behind the shoulders when driving the bar upward.

VARIATION

Dumbbell Incline Bench Press

Using dumbbells instead of barbells allows the hands to move independently of one another, more closely mimicking the demands encountered while swimming. Separate movement of the hands also prevents the stronger arm from compensating for the weaker one when a barbell is used.

Dip (Chest Version)

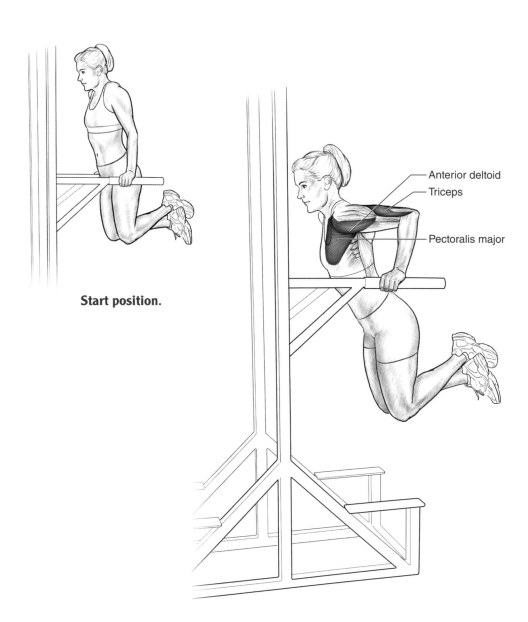

Start position.

Anterior deltoid

Triceps

Pectoralis major

Execution

1. Position yourself on a dip bar. Support your body weight with your elbows almost locked.
2. While lowering your chest downward, lean your upper body forward.
3. Stop when your upper arms are parallel to the floor or when you feel a stretch in the front part of the shoulders.
4. Push yourself upward until your elbows are almost locked.

Muscles Involved

Primary: Pectoralis major, triceps brachii, anterior deltoid

Secondary: None

Swimming Focus

This exercise targets both the pectoralis major and the triceps brachii, which will carry over to benefit all four strokes, contributing primarily to the pull phase. The exercise will be particularly useful to breaststrokers because it closely mimics the final portion of the underwater pull performed off the start and each turn wall. Depending on the angling of the torso, the focus of the exercise can be switched from the pectoralis major to the triceps brachii. Leaning forward will focus more on the pectoralis major, whereas maintaining a vertical, upright orientation of the chest will emphasize the triceps brachii.

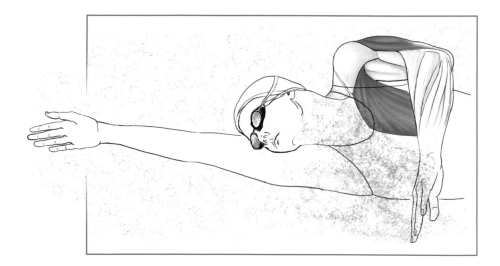

⚠️ **SAFETY TIP** When performing this exercise, do not let the shoulders drop below the elbows. Lower your body only until you feel a stretch in the front part of the shoulders. This exercise is best reserved for the early part of the season when yardage demands are low and the shoulders can handle the extra stress of the exercise. Young swimmer should avoid this exercise.

Standing Double-Arm Medicine Ball Throw Down

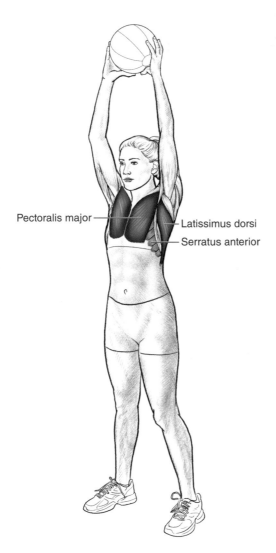

Pectoralis major

Latissimus dorsi

Serratus anterior

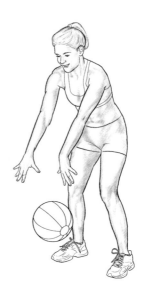

Finish position.

Execution

1. Using both hands, lift the medicine ball up over your head.
2. Forcefully throw the medicine ball downward, targeting a spot on the ground 1 foot (30 cm) in front of your feet.
3. Catch the medicine ball as it bounces up off the ground.

Muscles Involved

Primary: Pectoralis major, latissimus dorsi

Secondary: Serratus anterior

Swimming Focus

This exercise is one of the few that targets both the pectoralis major and latissimus dorsi in an explosive manner. It strengthens the initial portion of the pull phase for all four strokes, which is useful in making a quick transition from hand entry to a high-elbow position. Breaststrokers will find this exercise particularly beneficial because it is similar to the underwater pull that is performed off the start and each turn wall.

Keys to getting maximum benefit from the exercise begin with initiating the throw with the arms in an elongated position. This positioning will help ensure that the exercise is initiated with a tall, upright posture. A second key is making an explosive yet controlled throw and continuing the throw until you release the ball at the hips.

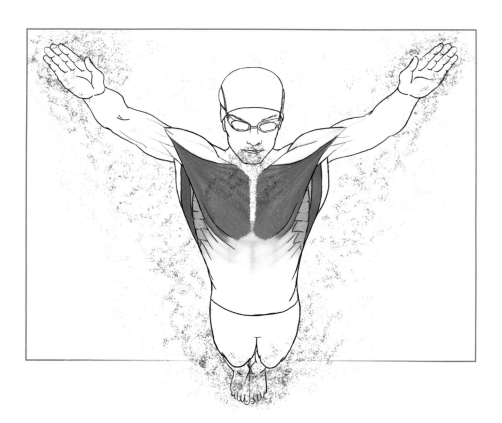

Supine Medicine Ball Partner Pass and Catch

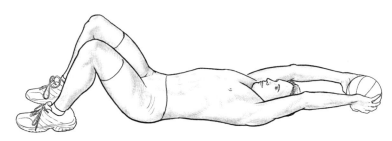

Start position.

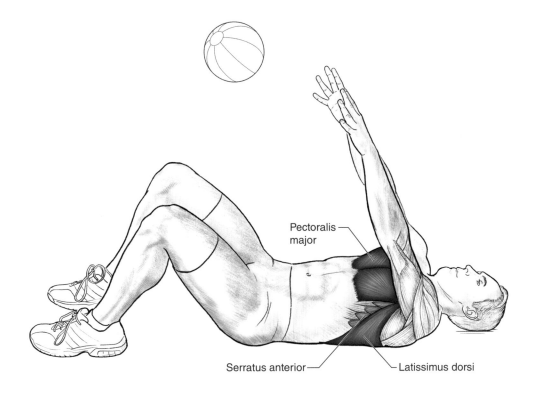

Pectoralis major

Serratus anterior

Latissimus dorsi

Execution

1. Lie on the ground with your knees bent and feet flat on ground.
2. Have your partner stand 4 to 5 feet (120 to 150 cm) away, out past your feet.
3. From an overhead position, forcefully throw the medicine ball to your partner, releasing it as your hands pass shoulder level.
4. Allow your hands to follow through until they are by your side.

Muscles Involved

Primary: Pectoralis major, latissimus dorsi

Secondary: Serratus anterior

Swimming Focus

Similar to the standing double-arm medicine ball throw down, this exercise targets both the pectoralis major and latissimus dorsi in an explosive manner. The primary difference between the two exercises is the release point of the medicine ball. In this exercise the medicine ball is released as the hands pass the shoulders. The main benefit of the exercise is that it strengthens both the pectoralis major and latissimus dorsi in an overhead position. This benefit will enhance your confidence and strength during the initial portion of the pull phase for all strokes.

A key to maximizing the benefits of the exercise is to initiate the throw with the arms in an elongated position. You can accentuate this positioning by catching the medicine ball passed to you by your partner, decelerating the ball, and then quickly reversing its direction to initiate the throwing motion.

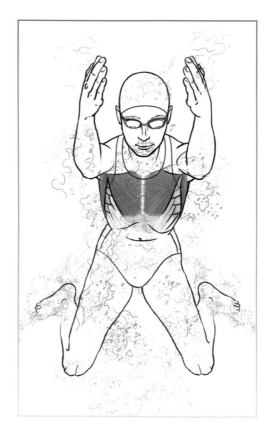

Wheelbarrow

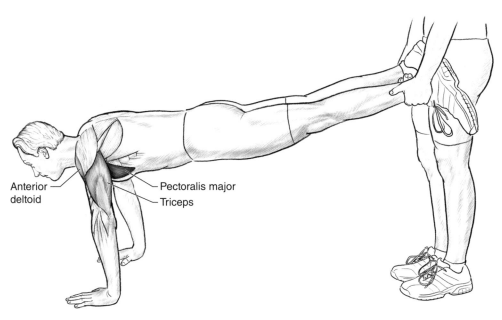

Anterior deltoid

Pectoralis major

Triceps

Execution

1. From a push-up position, have your partner grab both feet and lift them to waist level.
2. Focus on holding your body in a straight line from your ankles to the top of your head.
3. Moving one hand at a time, walk your hands forward.

Muscles Involved

Primary: Pectoralis major

Secondary: Anterior deltoid, triceps brachii

Swimming Focus

The wheelbarrow exercise focuses on several areas that are beneficial to the swimmer. As a strengthening exercise it targets the pectoralis major and triceps brachii, which are vital contributors to the portion of the pulling phase of all four strokes. The exercise also requires activation of the shoulder-, core-, and hip-stabilizing musculature, which will help with injury prevention and maintenance of a streamlined body position in the water. One of the biggest advantages of the wheelbarrow exercise is that it builds mental toughness.

The emphasis should be on maintaining the body in a straight line from the ankles to the tip of the head. Flaws encountered when performing this exercise include not holding the head in line with the rest of the body and allowing excessive arching or sagging of the back. Both alterations in body position increase the risk of injury. To transition into performing the exercise, first attempt to hold the wheelbarrow position without moving your hands. When you are able to hold this position with good technique for 60 seconds, you can begin to start the walking motion with your hands.

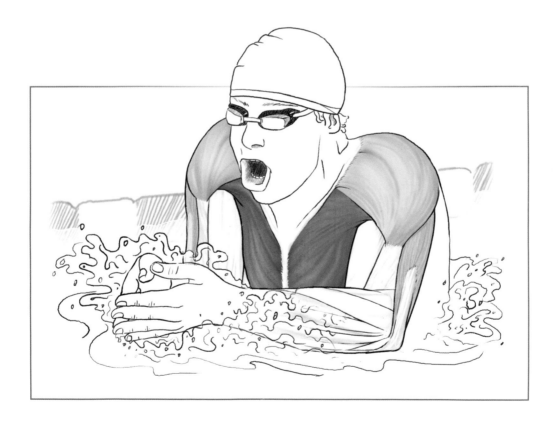

⚠ **SAFETY TIP** When performing this exercise on a pool deck, wear protective gloves to avoid unnecessary trauma to the hands.

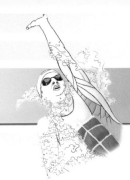

ABDOMEN

To move your body efficiently through the water, a coordinated movement of the arms and legs must occur. The key to this coordinated movement is a strong core, of which the muscles of the abdominal wall are a primary component. Besides helping to link the movement of the upper and lower body, the abdominal muscles assist with the body-rolling movements that take place during freestyle and backstroke and are responsible for the undulating movements of the torso that take place during butterfly, breaststroke, and underwater dolphin kicking.

The abdominal wall is composed of four paired muscles that extend from the rib cage to the pelvis. The muscles can be divided into two groups—a single anterior group and two lateral groups that mirror each other. The anterior group contains only one paired muscle, the rectus abdominis, which is divided into a right and left half by the midline of the body. The two lateral groups each contain a side of the remaining three paired muscles—the external oblique, internal oblique, and transversus abdominis (figure 5.1). In human motion and athletics, the abdominal muscles serve two primary functions: (1) movement, specifically forward trunk flexion (curling the trunk forward), lateral trunk flexion (bending to the side), and trunk rotation; and (2) stabilization of the low back and trunk. The motions mentioned earlier result from the coordinated activation of multiple muscle groups or the activation of a single muscle group.

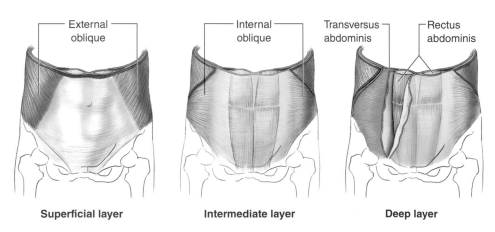

Superficial layer   **Intermediate layer**   **Deep layer**

Figure 5.1 Abdominal muscles.

The rectus abdominis, popularly known as the six pack, attaches superiorly to the sternum and the surrounding cartilage of ribs 5 through 7. The fibers then run vertically to attach to the middle of the pelvis at the pubic symphysis and pubic crest. The six-pack appearance results because the muscle is divided by and encased in a sheath of tissue called a fascia. The visible line running along the midline of the body dividing the muscle in two halves is known as the linea alba. Contraction of the upper fibers of the rectus abdominis curls the upper trunk downward, whereas contraction of the lower fibers pulls the pelvis upward toward the chest. Combined contraction of both the upper and lower fibers rolls the trunk into a ball.

The muscles of the two lateral groups are arranged into three layers. The external oblique forms the most superficial layer. From its attachment on the external surface of ribs 5 through 12, the fibers run obliquely (diagonally) to attach at the midline of the body along the linea alba and pelvis. If you were to think of your fingers as the fibers of this muscle, the fibers would run in the same direction as your fingers do when you put your hand into the front pocket of a pair of pants. Unilateral (single-sided) contraction of the muscle results in trunk rotation to the opposite side, meaning that contraction of the right external oblique rotates the trunk to the left. Bilateral contraction results in trunk flexion.

The next layer is formed by the internal oblique. The orientation of its fibers is perpendicular to those of the external oblique. This muscle originates from the upper part of the pelvis and from a structure known as the thoracolumbar fascia, which is a broad band of dense connective tissue that attaches to the spine in the upper- and lower-back region. From its posterior attachment, the internal oblique wraps around to the front of the abdomen, inserting at the linea alba and pubis. Unilateral contraction rotates the trunk to the same side, and bilateral contraction leads to trunk flexion. The deepest of the three layers is formed by the transversus abdominis, so named because the muscle fibers run transversely (horizontally) across the abdomen. The transversus abdominis arises from the internal surface of the cartilage of ribs 5 through 12, the upper part of pelvis, and the thoracolumbar fascia. The muscle joins with the internal oblique to attach along the midline of the body at the linea alba and pubis. Contraction of the transversus abdominis does not result in significant trunk motion, but it does join the other muscles of the lateral group to function as a core stabilizer. An analogy that often helps people grasp the core-stabilizing function of the muscles of the lateral group is to think of them as a corset that, when tightened, holds the core in a stabilized position.

Note that other muscles, including the serratus anterior and hip flexors, can be recruited along with the abdominal muscles when many of the exercises in this chapter are performed. The serratus anterior commonly functions as a stabilizer of the scapula, as described in chapter 3, but it is also activated during many of the exercises that target the external and internal obliques. The two primary hip flexors are the rectus femoris and the iliopsoas. As described in chapter 7, these muscles can either flex the hip or flex the lower trunk, depending on whether the lower extremity or trunk is stabilized.

The role of the core abdominal muscles in swimming can be easily broken down according to their roles as trunk flexors, trunk rotators, and trunk stabilizers. Through their ability to flex the trunk, the rectus abdominis, external oblique, and internal oblique all play important roles in the movements that take place during swimming. For example, flexion of the trunk during flip turns is initiated by the upper fibers of the rectus abdominis, sustained by the lower fibers of the rectus abdominis, and helped to completion by both obliques. The trunk flexors are also important contributors to the wavelike, or undulating, body roll that takes place during butterfly, breaststroke, and underwater dolphin kicking. Besides contributing to flexion of the trunk, the obliques are responsible for trunk rotational movements. Strong obliques are vital to enhancing the speed of open turns performed during butterfly and breaststroke. The obliques are active during the body-rolling movements that take place during freestyle and backstroke, functioning to link the movements of the arms with the movements of the hips and legs. As previously mentioned, through their ability to function like a corset, the abdominal muscles are central to stabilizing the trunk. Trunk stability is one of the keys to efficient movement through the water, because it ensures a firm base of support upon which the arms and legs can generate their propulsive forces.

When incorporating abdominal strengthening exercises into the dryland program, you must understand the importance of focusing on correct technique. The focal point of correct technique begins with the conscious recruitment of the abdominal muscles, often referred to as setting, or locking in, the core, as described in the sidebar on page 13 of chapter 2. Setting the core first involves using the abdominal muscles to control the positioning of the hips and low back. This is best done by lying on the back, as pictured in the starting position for the first exercise of this chapter, the hollow hold. In this position, contraction of the abdominal muscles rolls the hips backward, pressing the low back against the floor. Conversely, contraction of the hip flexors rolls the hips forward, causing the low back to arch. After becoming comfortable with rolling the hips forward and backward, attention should be switched to holding the low back and pelvis in a neutral, fixed position. A useful approach to maintaining this neutral position is to visualize all the abdominal muscles as a corset and to focus consciously on contracting the abdominal muscles in this manner. You should perform the process of setting the core at the start of every abdominal exercise, and it should remain the underlying focus while you execute the entire exercise. The most common indicators that you are not setting the core are excessive arching of the low back and, if you are performing an exercise while facing the ground, excessive rounding of the low back and the hips rising toward the ceiling. Either of these compensatory movements is an indication that you are relying on your stronger hip flexors (rectus femoris and iliopsoas) to hold the body position instead of your abdominal musculature.

Hollow Hold

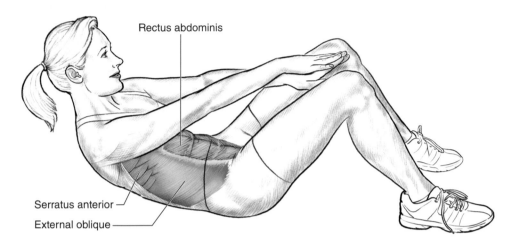

Rectus abdominis

Serratus anterior

External oblique

Execution

1. Lie face up on the floor with your arms by your sides, knees bent, and feet on the floor.
2. Tighten the abdominal muscles like a corset to set your core.
3. Lift your shoulders 6 inches (15 cm) off the ground, making sure to keep the low back in a stable and fixed position.
4. While lifting the shoulders, reach your arms toward the tops of your knees.
5. Hold this position for 60 seconds or until you are unable to keep the low back in the set position.

Muscles Involved

Primary: Rectus abdominis (upper fibers)

Secondary: External oblique, internal oblique, transversus abdominis, serratus anterior

Swimming Focus

This exercise is a good way to learn how to use your abdominal musculature to position the hips for correct technique and to stabilize the low back. In the starting position, you can experiment with contracting and relaxing your abdominal musculature to roll your hips forward and backward. Practicing these movements will help you gain a feel for the positioning of your hips. Gaining this feel will help you detect when you haven fallen out of the proper positioning for the exercise. A partner can monitor your positioning by testing whether he or she can slide a hand under your low back. If your partner can slide a whole hand under your low back, then you have fallen out of the proper position. When you lift your shoulders off the ground, look down your arms and past your knees to increase recruitment of the upper fibers of the rectus abdominis.

Direct benefits include strengthening of the core musculature, which will carry over to a tighter streamline and a reduction in the risk of injury. By targeting the upper fibers of the rectus abdominis, this exercise helps with the initiation of trunk flexion during freestyle and backstroke flip turns.

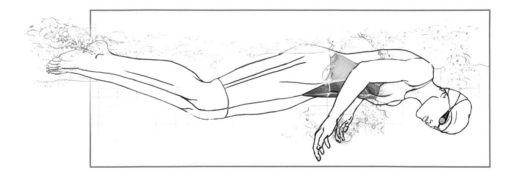

VARIATION

Hollow Hold With Feet Elevated

Incorporation of the legs will make the exercise significantly more challenging. Again, the key to performing the exercise properly is maintaining contact between the low back and the ground.

Watch TV

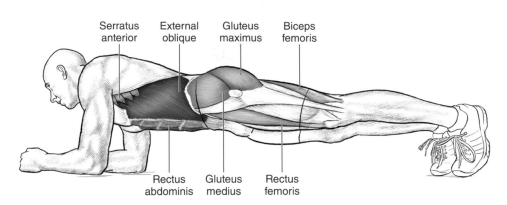

Serratus anterior · External oblique · Gluteus maximus · Biceps femoris · Rectus abdominis · Gluteus medius · Rectus femoris

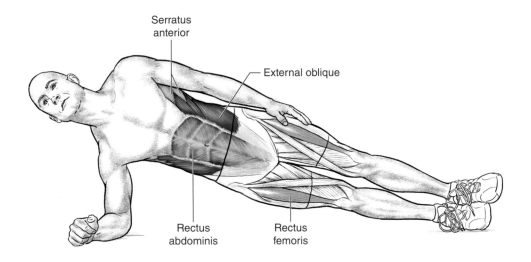

Serratus anterior · External oblique · Rectus abdominis · Rectus femoris

Execution

1. Facedown, support your body weight on your toes and forearms.
2. After holding the starting position for 15 seconds, rotate your body so that it is perpendicular to the floor and supported by one arm.
3. Hold this position for 15 seconds and then rotate back to the starting position.
4. Next, rotate your body so that it is again perpendicular to the floor but now facing the opposite direction. Hold for 15 seconds.

Muscles Involved

Primary: Rectus abdominis, external oblique, internal oblique, transversus abdominis

Secondary: Serratus anterior, rectus femoris, gluteus maximus, gluteus medius, biceps femoris, semitendinosus, semimembranosus

Swimming Focus

This exercise is a good way to transition from the hollow hold to a more challenging exercise when the primary focus is engaging the abdominal musculature to stabilize the low back. Again, monitoring the positioning of the hips and low back is important when performing the exercise. In both the starting and the ending position, the body should be held in a straight line from the ankles all the way to the tip of the head. If the hips begin to drop, the swimmer should be cued to focus on tightening the abdominal musculature. Monitoring the position of the head is also important because its position will indirectly affect the positioning of the low back. If the head is out of alignment with the rest of the body, holding proper body positioning will be much more challenging. As you become more proficient at performing the exercise, gradually increase the amount of time that you spend in each position. The goal is to reach 30 to 45 seconds.

This is an excellent all-around exercise for learning how to engage the abdominal muscles in a manner that will carry over to better maintenance of proper hip and low back positioning during all four strokes and when streamlining off starts and turns.

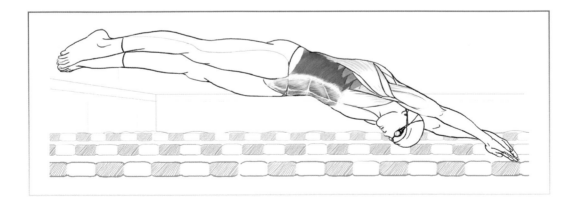

V-Up

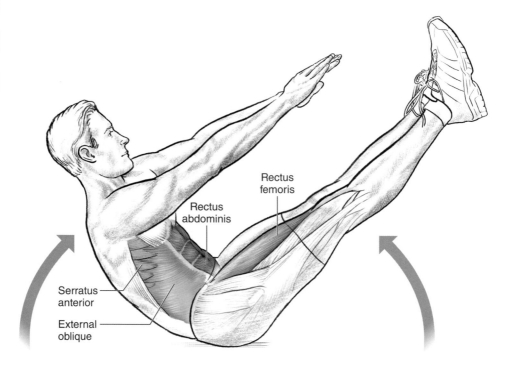

Execution

1. Lying face up in a streamlined position, stabilize your core by tightening the abdominal musculature.

2. In unison, bring your arms forward and lift your legs until your hands are able to touch your feet.

3. Slowly reverse the movement, stopping when your hands and feet are just above the ground. Then repeat.

Muscles Involved

Primary: Rectus abdominis (upper and lower fibers)

Secondary: External oblique, internal oblique, transversus abdominis, serratus anterior, rectus femoris, iliopsoas

Swimming Focus

This exercise targets and strengthens the rectus abdominis through a wide range of motion, making it a useful exercise for freestylers or backstroke swimmers who are trying to improve the speed of their flip turns. Emphasizing the tight streamlined position after each repetition will benefit all strokes. When initiating the movement, avoid swinging your hands up and down to generate momentum; this is a form of cheating. The exercise can be made more challenging by holding the streamlined position with the hands and feet just off the ground for 3 to 4 seconds after each repetition.

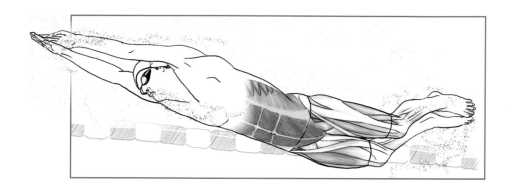

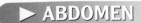

Flutter Kicks

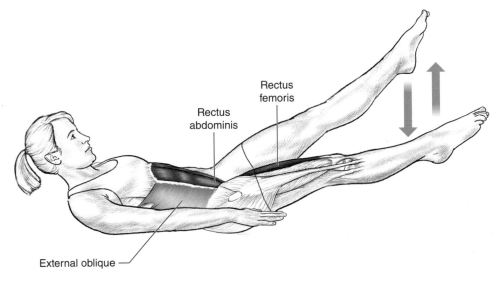

Execution

1. Lie on the floor with your arms at your sides and tighten the abdominal muscles to set your core.

2. Lift your shoulders 4 inches (10 cm) off the ground and your feet 12 inches (30 cm) off the ground, making sure to keep the low back in a neutral position.

3. Hold this position and flutter kick for 60 seconds or until you are unable to keep the low back stabilized in a neutral position.

Muscles Involved

Primary: Rectus abdominis (lower fibers), rectus femoris

Secondary: External oblique, internal oblique, transversus abdominis, iliopsoas

Swimming Focus

This is a good exercise to transition to after mastering the hollow hold. As with the hollow hold, the main emphasis should be on keeping the low back in a stable and fixed position. If the low back begins to arch, the abdominal musculature is no longer holding the low back in a stable and fixed position and is being overpowered by the hip flexors. Incorporation of the flutter-kicking motion makes this exercise particularly useful to freestyle and backstroke swimmers.

To avoid relying on the hands to hold the upper body in its curled position, perform this exercise by holding your hands 1 inch (2.5 cm) off the ground.

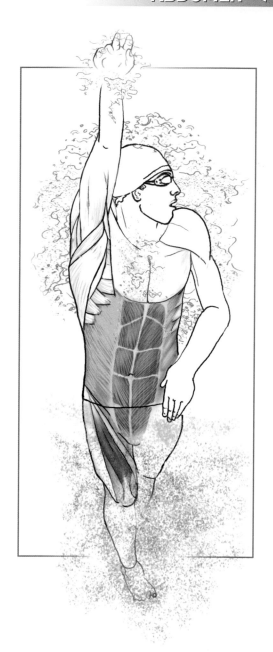

VARIATION

Streamlined Flutter Kicks

A variation is to hold your arms in an overhead streamlined position. This variation increases the difficulty of the exercise and makes it more specific to swimmers. Because of the increased difficulty, be sure to keep your focus on holding the core tight and maintaining the low back in a neutral position.

Physioball Crunch

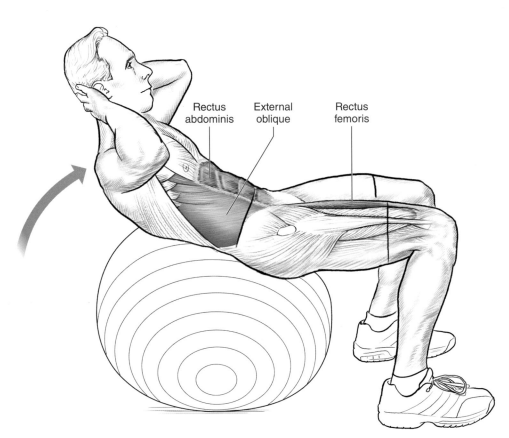

Rectus abdominis

External oblique

Rectus femoris

Execution

1. Begin in a bridge position with the ball positioned in the middle of your back. Your fingers should be touching but not interlocked behind your head.

2. Raise your shoulders toward the ceiling and bring your chest forward in a crunching motion.

3. Slowly lower your shoulders back to the starting position.

Muscles Involved

Primary: Rectus abdominis

Secondary: External oblique, internal oblique, transversus abdominis, rectus femoris

Swimming Focus

Because the movement begins with the back in an extended position, this exercise strengthens the rectus abdominis through a range of motion not targeted by any of the other exercises listed in this chapter. This feature makes it a valuable exercise for both breaststroke and butterfly swimmers because it contributes to the undulating body movements that occur during both of these strokes.

While performing the exercise, keep your fingers loose behind your head and do not pull your head forward with your hands. Additionally, the positioning of your body on the physioball should remain constant during the entire exercise. If your hips roll back, your shoulders will rise and you will lose the isolation of the abdominal muscles. An easy way to prevent this from happening is to focus on keeping the thighs parallel to the ground.

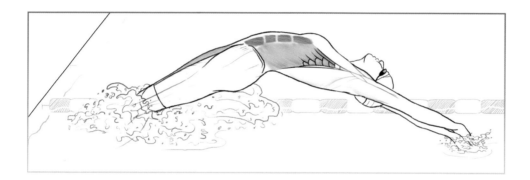

VARIATION

Physioball Crunch With Trunk Rotation

Incorporation of the twisting motion diverts the focus of this exercise from the rectus abdominis to the internal and external obliques. This exercise is useful in linking the movement of the arms to the movement of the legs in freestyle and backstroke.

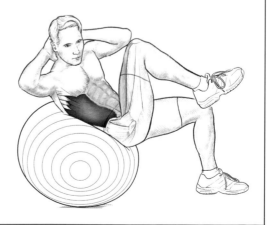

Cable Crunch

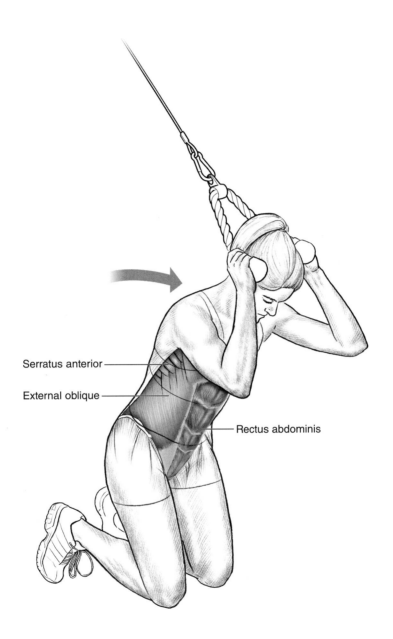

Serratus anterior

External oblique

Rectus abdominis

Execution

1. Kneel on the ground in front of a pulley machine. With your elbows bent, hold the separate ends of a rope pulley handle behind your head.

2. Holding your hips stationary, bend at the waist and crunch your torso downward.

3. Slowly return to the starting position.

Muscles Involved

Primary: Rectus abdominis

Secondary: Serratus anterior, internal oblique, external oblique, transversus abdominis

Swimming Focus

Use of the pulley machine allows this exercise to be performed with variable resistance. As a result, the focus of the exercise can be shifted from endurance to strength simply by altering the weight and number of repetitions performed. The variable resistance offers an advantage when compared with most of the exercises in this chapter, which depend primarily on body weight. The motion performed during the exercise closely mimics the motion performed during a flip turn, but because of the wide range of motion through which the abdominal muscles are targeted and the variable resistance, this exercise is beneficial across all four strokes.

To gain maximal benefit when performing the exercise, emphasize a curling motion, beginning with the upper torso and continuing all the way down to the waistline. When performing the exercise, resist the temptation to pull downward with the hands. Doing this shifts the focus away from the abdominal muscles and places unnecessary stress on the joints and muscles of the neck.

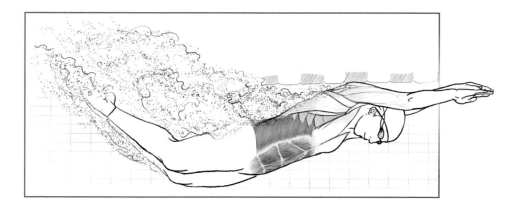

Seated Physioball Abdominal Hold

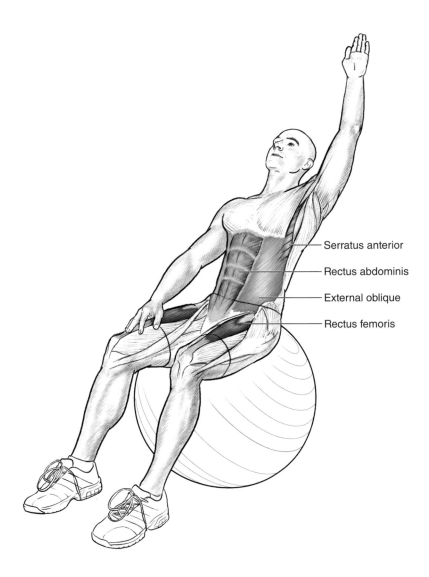

Serratus anterior

Rectus abdominis

External oblique

Rectus femoris

Execution

1. In an upright seated position on a physioball, set your abdominal muscles.
2. Slowly lean backward until your upper torso is at a 45-degree angle to the floor.
3. Lift one arm forward until it is in a streamlined position.
4. Lower and then repeat with the opposite arm.

Muscles Involved

Primary: Rectus abdominis, rectus femoris, iliopsoas

Secondary: Serratus anterior, internal oblique, external oblique, transversus abdominis

Swimming Focus

It is easy to visualize how this exercise can contribute directly to strengthening the core stabilizers as they are used while swimming backstroke. The addition of trunk rotational movements similar to those performed while swimming backstroke emphasizes the internal and external obliques. By moving both arms in unison and holding a streamlined position, the focus of the exercise shifts to strengthening the core muscles as they contribute to maintaining a streamline during both starts and turns.

While performing this exercise, the main focus must be placed on (1) maintaining the set abdominal position during the entire exercise and (2) performing the arm and trunk movements in a slow, controlled manner.

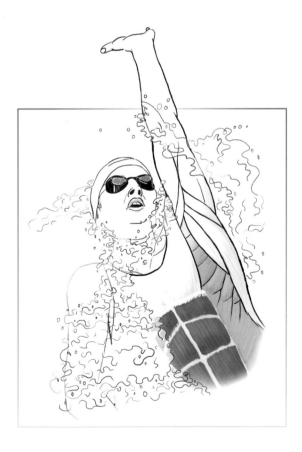

Russian Twist

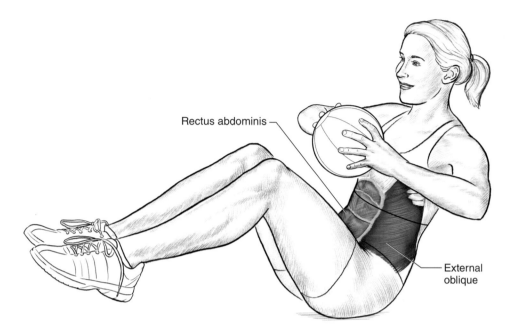

Rectus abdominis

External oblique

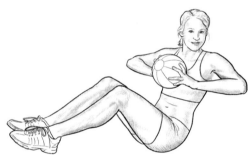

Finish position.

Execution

1. From a seated bent-knee position, tighten your abdominal muscles, lean backward, and lift your feet 4 to 6 inches (10 to 15 cm) off the ground. Hold a medicine ball in your hands at your chest.

2. Moving only with your trunk, rotate to one side. Quickly reverse the movement and rotate to the opposite side.

3. Continue until you have completed the set number of repetitions.

Muscles Involved

Primary: Rectus abdominis, external oblique, internal oblique

Secondary: Psoas major

Swimming Focus

The main focus of this exercise is the internal and external obliques, which are extremely important in linking the movements of the arms and legs during freestyle and backstroke, especially when you are in an elongated position. The upper-trunk rotational movements are similar to those performed during open turns for both butterfly and breaststroke, so this exercise can also be used to improve the speed at which you can complete a turn and get off the wall.

To keep the focus of the exercise on the abdominal musculature, hold the medicine ball close to the chest. If you hold the ball away from your chest and emphasize touching it to the ground, you may compensate by using the shoulder muscles instead of the abdominal muscles.

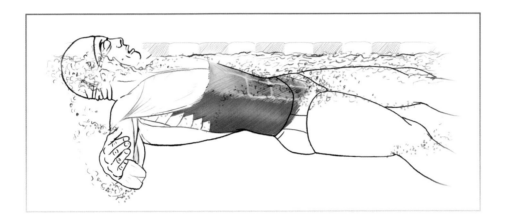

Kneeling Chop

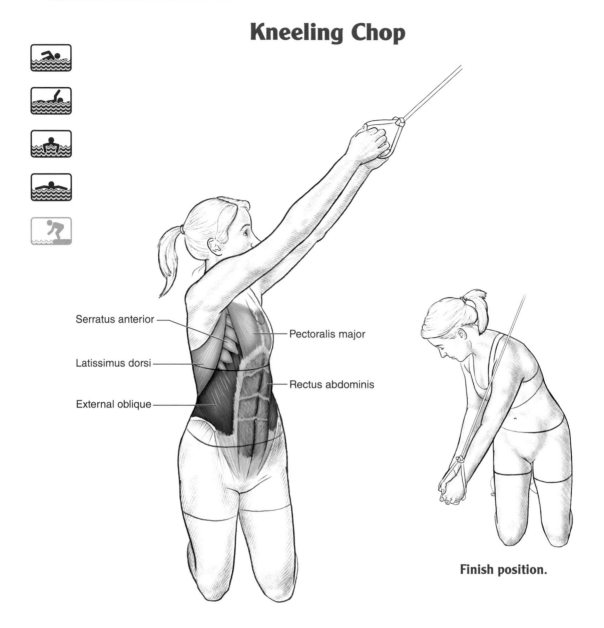

Serratus anterior

Pectoralis major

Latissimus dorsi

Rectus abdominis

External oblique

Finish position.

Execution

1. Position yourself so that when you are kneeling, the high pulley is diagonally behind your shoulder.
2. Reaching up and back, grasp the handle with both hands.
3. Initiate the movement with your abdominal muscles. The arms should act as an extension of the torso.
4. Using an arcing movement, guide the handle downward toward the opposite knee.
5. Reverse the movement to return to the starting position.

Muscles Involved

Primary: Rectus abdominis, external oblique, internal oblique

Secondary: Serratus anterior, latissimus dorsi, pectoralis major

Swimming Focus

Because it starts with the arms and trunk in an elongated and stretched position, this exercise helps swimmers develop confidence and strength in their stroke during the initial portion of the pulling phase of all four strokes. Another key to this exercise is that the actions performed recruit the latissimus dorsi and pectoralis major, which helps to link their activation with that of the involved abdominal muscles. This coordination in muscle activation helps swimmers generate more power with their arm movements by linking them to the core.

When performing the exercise, the head should follow the movements of the hands. This action links the movements of the arms to the movements of the torso, which in turn targets the abdominal muscles. Not doing this poses the risk that the movements will be performed predominantly with the arms rather than the trunk, thus negating most of the benefits of the exercise.

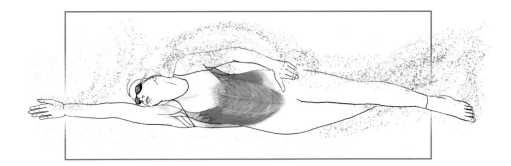

Physioball Prayer Roll

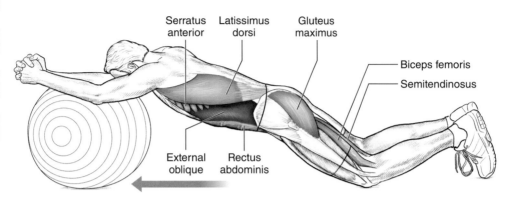

Execution

1. Using your forearms, support your upper body on a physioball. Support your lower body with your knees and toes.
2. Set your abdominal muscles to stabilize your spine in a neutral position.
3. Roll the ball out slowly, allowing your arms to move with the ball and your knees to straighten.
4. Pause in the ending position and then return to the start.

Muscles Involved

Primary: Rectus abdominis, external oblique, internal oblique, transversus abdominis

Secondary: Latissimus dorsi, serratus anterior, gluteus maximus, biceps femoris, semitendinosus, semimembranosus

Swimming Focus

This core-strengthening exercise is particularly useful for breaststrokers. It can help them develop confidence when the body is in an elongated position at the start of the pulling phase. Additionally, the exercise targets the abdominal muscles in a way that will carry over to strengthening the undulating body movements that occur during breaststroke and butterfly.

To get the maximum benefit out of performing this exercise, you must stabilize the spine in a neutral position for the entire time. Dropping the hips and arching the back is a sign that this control has been lost. The difficulty of the exercise can be modified by altering the starting forearm placement on the physioball. If the starting position of the hand and forearms is lower on the ball and closer to the floor, the exercise becomes more difficult because you will be able to roll the ball farther away from the body.

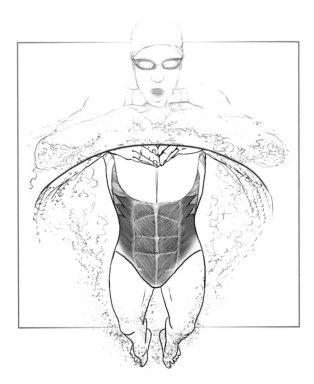

Physioball Upper-Trunk Rotation

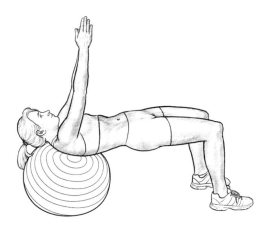

Start position.

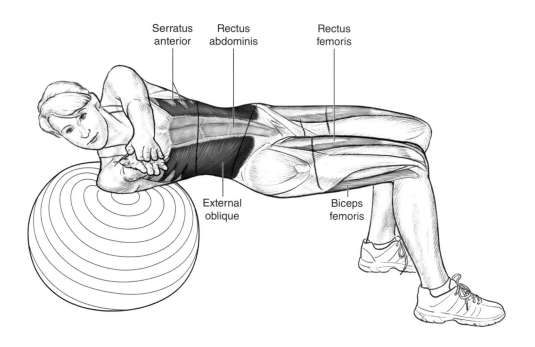

Serratus anterior — Rectus abdominis — Rectus femoris — External oblique — Biceps femoris

Execution

1. Sit on a physioball and slide down into a bridge position with your neck and shoulders balanced on the ball. Point your arms toward the ceiling.

2. While keeping your hips straight and your spine in a neutral position, rotate your upper body to one side.

3. Pause and then rotate to the opposite side.

Muscles Involved

Primary: External oblique, internal oblique, transversus abdominis

Secondary: Serratus anterior, rectus abdominis, rectus femoris, gluteus maximus, biceps femoris, semitendinosus, semimembranosus

Swimming Focus

The rotational movements performed during the exercise are useful for strengthening the oblique muscles, which in turn will help to strengthen the linkage between the legs and arms during freestyle and backstroke. This exercise also improves awareness and control of hip position, which can help a swimmer who is having trouble keeping the hips elevated when swimming backstroke.

The degree of rotational movement performed during the exercise depends on the ability to keep the hips straight, meaning that the shoulders should be rotated until the hip position can no longer be controlled. When just learning how to perform the exercise or for those with weak core musculature, the best approach is to keep the rotational movements small and focus initially on maintaining the bridge position for a 60-second hold. As proficiency with the exercise increases, the focus can be shifted toward increasing the rotational movements of the upper body and performing a set number of repetitions.

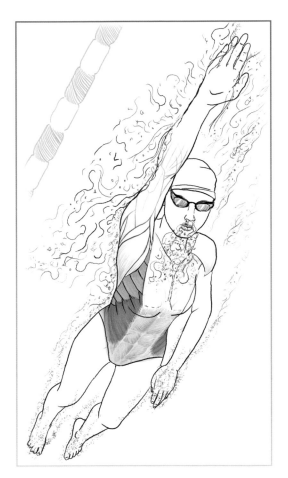

Physioball Jackknife

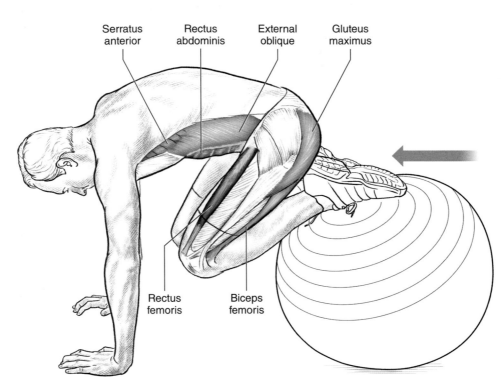

Serratus anterior — Rectus abdominis — External oblique — Gluteus maximus

Rectus femoris — Biceps femoris

Execution

1. Begin with a physioball positioned under your feet, and then walk your hands out to move into the starting position.

2. When you are in the starting position, focus on holding your legs and body in a straight line from your ankles to the top of your head.

3. Initiate a curling motion with your abdominal muscles and pull your knees up to your chest.

4. Pause at the ending position and then reverse the leg movement.

Muscles Involved

Primary: Rectus abdominis, rectus femoris, iliopsoas

Secondary: Serratus anterior, external oblique, internal oblique, gluteus maximus, biceps femoris, semitendinosus, semimembranosus

Swimming Focus

For many swimmers, simply attaining the starting position for this exercise will be a challenge. The initial emphasis should be on holding the body in a straight line from the feet to the tip of the head for a 60-second duration. Developing the strength to hold this position will greatly enhance your ability to hold a tight streamlined position in the water. Incorporating the trunk-curling motion with hip flexion shifts the focus of this exercise from a general stabilizing exercise to one that targets the rectus abdominis and the hip flexors (rectus femoris and iliopsoas). As a result of this combined strengthening, this exercise strengthens the relationship between the core musculature and the hip flexors, which enhances the hip-rolling movements that take place in breaststroke and butterfly.

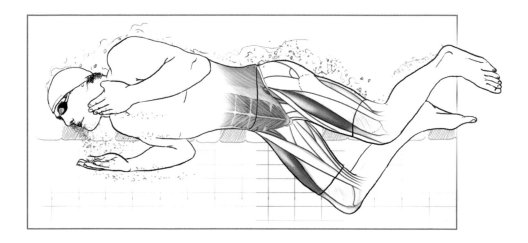

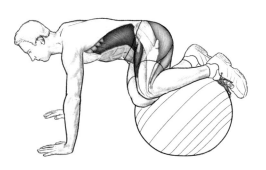

VARIATION

Physioball Jackknife With Twist

The addition of the twisting motion shifts the focus from the rectus abdominis to the internal and external obliques. This alteration broadens the benefits of the exercise, making it useful to freestyle and backstroke swimmers.

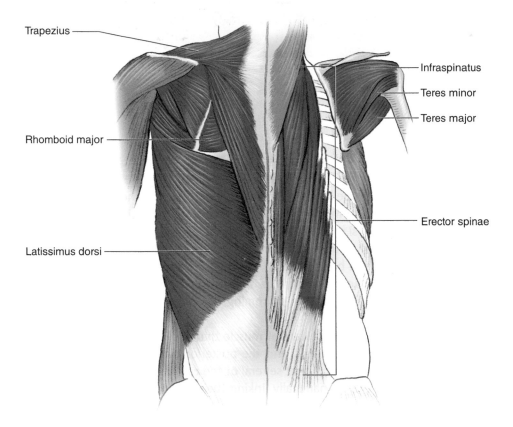

Trapezius

Infraspinatus

Teres minor

Teres major

Rhomboid major

Erector spinae

Latissimus dorsi

Figure 6.1   Back muscles.

one muscle group contracts, lateral flexion (side bending) and rotation of the trunk occur to the side of the muscle group that is contracting. The gluteus maximus and the hamstring muscle group (biceps femoris, semitendinosus, and semimembranosus) are commonly activated in unison with the erector spinae because they extend the hip, a movement that commonly takes place in conjunction with extension of the spine; their anatomy will be discussed in chapter 7.

Although the pectoralis major and the latissimus dorsi are both defined as humeral propellers and together produce most of the upper-extremity propulsive forces responsible for driving a swimmer through the water, of the two, the latissimus dorsi is the prime mover. During freestyle, butterfly, and breaststroke, the latissimus dorsi begins contributing shortly after hand entry at the initiation of the propulsive portion of the pulling phase. During backstroke, no delay occurs in the activation of the latissimus dorsi. In all four stokes the latissimus dorsi remains active from its point of recruitment during the propulsive phase until the initiation of the recovery phase. In butterfly, it contributes to the initiation of the recovery phase. For every exercise that primarily targets the lats, extra emphasis should be placed on pinching the shoulder blades together in the ending position. Doing this increases the recruitment of the musculature that stabilizes the shoulder blades, further increasing the benefit of the exercise.

The erector spinae muscle group is extremely important in maintaining proper horizontal body alignment in the water, especially during backstroke. Whenever a swimmer has difficulty holding a tight streamline in the water or allows the hips to drop while swimming backstroke, the erector spinae should be near the top of the list of suspected areas of weakness. The erector spinae muscle group produces the extension of the spine that takes place with the undulating body movements performed with underwater dolphin kicking, butterfly, and breaststroke. The erector spinae muscle group also plays a vital role in the starting motion of all four strokes. During starts performed from the blocks, it is one of the primary muscle groups responsible for creating the streamlined body position. During backstroke starts, contraction of the erector spinae leads to the arching motion that allows the swimmer to get off the wall and into the water quickly.

Chin-Up

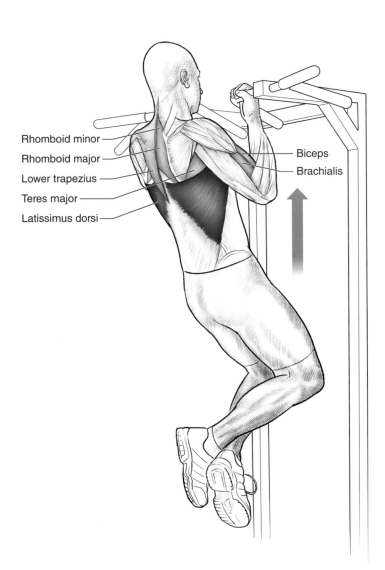

Rhomboid minor
Rhomboid major
Lower trapezius
Teres major
Latissimus dorsi

Biceps
Brachialis

Execution

1. Grasp the bar with an underhand grip, with the palms facing your body. Your hands should be slightly wider than shoulder-width apart. Hold your knees in a bent position and cross one foot over the other.

2. From a hanging position pull your body upward, focusing on bringing your chest to the bar.

3. Pause at the top of the movement and then slowly lower to a hanging position.

Muscles Involved

Primary: Latissimus dorsi

Secondary: Biceps brachii, brachialis, lower trapezius, rhomboid major, rhomboid minor, teres major

Swimming Focus

Chin-ups are a great addition to any dryland program because they can be done wherever a chin-up or pull-up bar is available. In comparison with the hand positioning for pull-ups, the hand placement for chin-ups emphasizes the elbow flexors (biceps brachii and brachialis). By targeting both the latissimus dorsi and the elbow flexors, this exercise benefits all swimmers by strengthening the pulling phase of their strokes. Because chin-ups are generally a challenging exercise for most swimmers, they are useful for building mental toughness. To help you reach your goal number of repetitions, a partner can assist by supporting your feet.

Make sure that your body movements are slow and controlled during the exercise. Excessive jerking and swinging of the legs is a form of cheating.

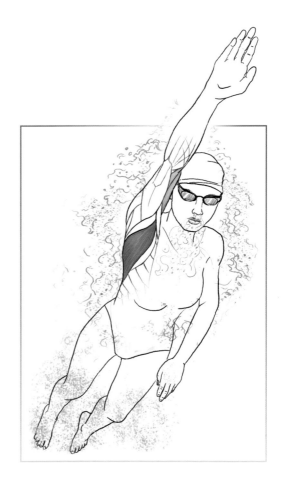

⚠ SAFETY TIP When returning to the starting position, lower your body in a controlled manner to avoid placing extra stress on the shoulders, which can occur if you allow your body to drop down quickly. Also, avoid hanging in the starting position for a prolonged period because doing this also places extra stress on the shoulders.

Pull-Up

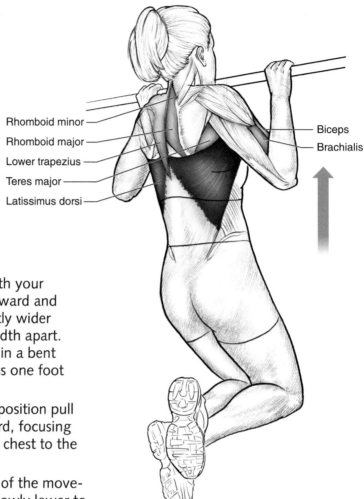

Rhomboid minor
Rhomboid major
Lower trapezius
Teres major
Latissimus dorsi

Biceps
Brachialis

Execution

1. Grasp the bar with your palms facing outward and your hands slightly wider than shoulder-width apart. Hold your knees in a bent position and cross one foot over the other.

2. From a hanging position pull your body upward, focusing on bringing your chest to the bar.

3. Pause at the top of the movement and then slowly lower to a hanging position.

Muscles Involved

Primary: Latissimus dorsi

Secondary: Lower trapezius, rhomboid major, rhomboid minor, teres major, biceps brachii, brachialis

⚠ **SAFETY TIP** When returning to the starting position, lower your body in a controlled manner to avoid placing extra stress on the shoulders, which can occur if you allow your body to drop down quickly. Also, avoid hanging in the starting position for a prolonged period because doing this also places extra stress on the shoulders.

Swimming Focus

Like chin-ups, pull-ups are easy to add to a dryland program because they can be performed almost anywhere. The hand positioning, opposite that used in chin-ups (palms facing away instead of toward the body), decreases the emphasis on the elbow flexors but is more similar to the hand positioning used during the four competitive strokes. This exercise strengthens the muscles responsible for the initial portion of the pull phase by targeting the latissimus dorsi with the arms in an overhead and elongated position. The difficult nature of the exercise builds mental toughness. To help you reach your goal number of repetitions, a partner can assist by supporting your feet.

Jerking body movements and swinging of the legs at the start of the movement are discouraged because they are a form of cheating.

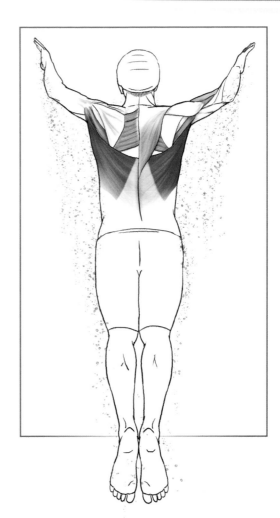

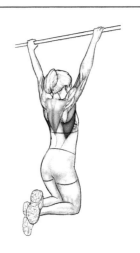

VARIATION

Wide-Grip Pull-Up

The wider positioning of the hands gears the exercise more toward breaststroke and butterfly swimmers who are trying to increase the strength of the midportion of the pulling phase.

Lat Pull-Down

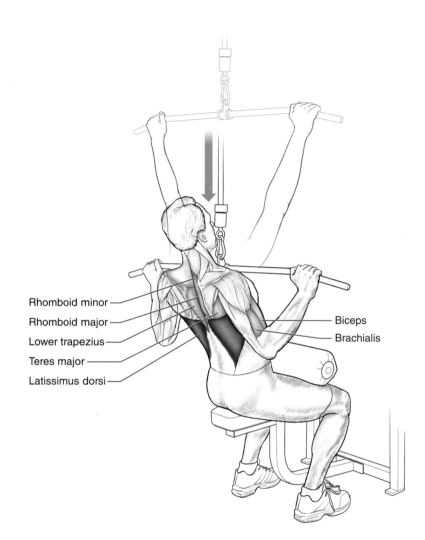

Rhomboid minor
Rhomboid major
Lower trapezius
Teres major
Latissimus dorsi

Biceps
Brachialis

Execution

1. Sit at the machine and use an overhand grip. Position your hands on the bar 6 to 8 inches (15 to 20 cm) wider than the width of your shoulders.
2. Pull the bar down to your upper chest, arching your back slightly.
3. Focus on tightening your lats and pinching your shoulder blades together.
4. Slowly return to the starting position.

Muscles Involved

Primary: Latissimus dorsi

Secondary: Lower trapezius, rhomboid major, rhomboid minor, teres major, biceps brachii, brachialis

Swimming Focus

The lat pull-down is a good all-around exercise for targeting the latissimus dorsi and has a beneficial effect on the pulling phase of all four competitive strokes. Although the body movements performed are similar to those used in pull-ups, lat pull-downs offer the advantage that the resistance is variable and does not depend on body weight. When performing the exercise, focus on keeping your elbows high to mimic more closely the catch position of the pull phase. Although arching your back slightly when bringing the bar down to your chest is OK, avoid leaning backward and using your body weight instead of your latissimus dorsi to pull the weight down.

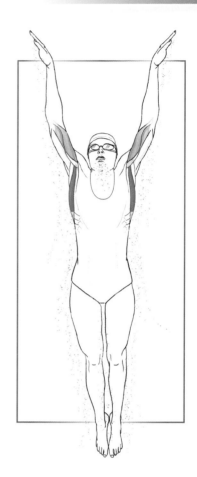

⚠ **SAFETY TIP** Perform the exercise as illustrated. The more traditional lat pull-down, in which the bar is brought behind the head to the base of the neck, places extra stress on the shoulder joints.

VARIATION

Single-Arm Lat Pull-Down

Isolating the exercise to one arm allows you to add a rotational trunk movement that more closely mimics the movements performed while swimming. Single-arm isolation also allows extra emphasis to be placed on scapular retraction.

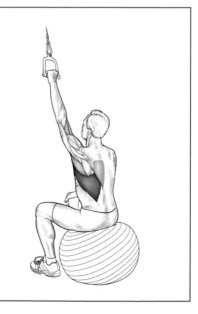

Standing Straight-Arm Pull-Down

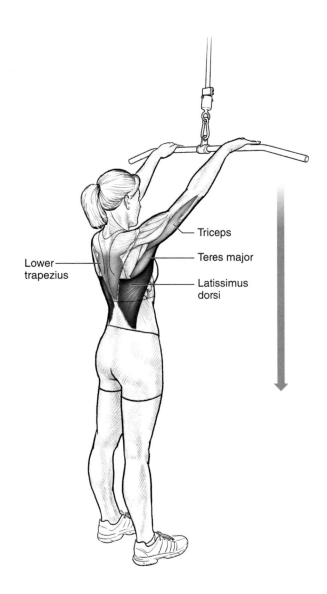

Triceps

Teres major

Lower trapezius

Latissimus dorsi

Execution

1. Stand facing the pulley machine. Using an overhand grip, position your hands slightly wider than the width of your shoulders.

2. Holding your elbows in 30 degrees of flexion, pull the bar down to your thighs in an arcing motion.

3. Bring the bar to within 1 inch (2.5 cm) of touching your thighs and then slowly return to the starting position.

Muscles Involved

Primary: Latissimus dorsi, pectoralis major

Secondary: Lower trapezius, teres major, triceps brachii

Swimming Focus

Similar to the lat pull-down, the standing straight-arm pull-down is beneficial for swimmers because the start of the exercise targets the latissimus dorsi in an overhead elongated position, thus strengthening the initial portion of the pulling phase. An added benefit of the straight-arm pull-down is that it takes the arms through a much larger range of motion than do chin-ups, pull-ups, and lat pull-downs. By helping to strengthen the muscles through the entire pulling motion, the exercise is more specific to the demands of swimming.

A key to isolating the latissimus dorsi during the exercise is to maintain the elbows in a fixed position and to keep the elbows high during the entire motion. Allowing the elbow position to change during the exercise shifts the demands of the exercise from the lats to the triceps brachii. Holding the torso still is also important. Bobbing or dipping of the torso is a form of cheating.

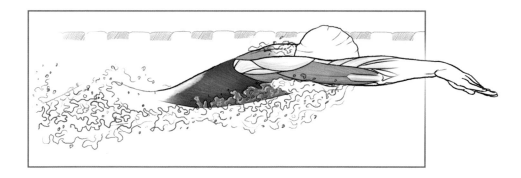

Double-Arm Seated Machine Row

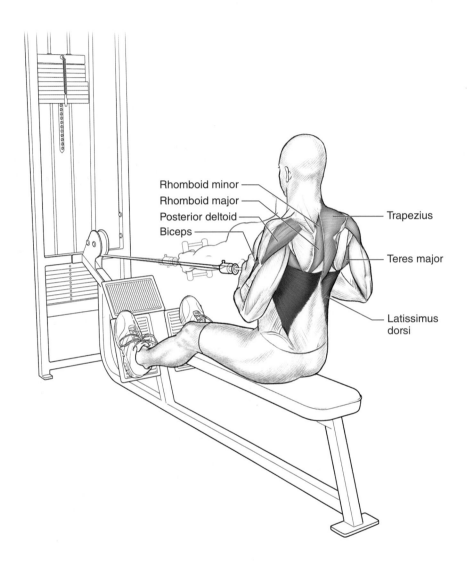

Rhomboid minor
Rhomboid major
Posterior deltoid
Biceps
Trapezius
Teres major
Latissimus dorsi

Execution

1. Sit on a bench facing a pulley machine. Grab the pulley handles so that your palms are facing each other.
2. Keeping your back perpendicular to the floor, pull the handles in toward your lower chest.
3. Pinch your shoulder blades together and pause in the ending position.
4. Return to the starting position by slowly lowering the weight.

Muscles Involved

Primary: Latissimus dorsi

Secondary: Trapezius, rhomboid major, rhomboid minor, teres major, posterior deltoid, biceps brachii

Swimming Focus

This exercise builds strength in the latissimus dorsi. It can be particularly beneficial to the breaststroker who wants to increase the strength of the latter half of the pull when the hands are brought together in the midline of the body. By targeting the secondary muscles, particularly the scapular retractors, the exercise enhances the scapular retraction that takes place during the final portion of the breaststroke pulling phase as well as the scapular retraction that is vital to an efficient recovery phase during butterfly. Strengthening of the scapular stabilizers also helps to stabilize the scapula, which generates a stronger base of support for the entire shoulder girdle.

Altering the weight used during the exercise shifts the emphasis to different muscles. Lighter weights allow a greater degree of scapular retraction, thus placing more focus on the rhomboid major, rhomboid minor, and trapezius. In contrast, increasing the weight places more demand on the latissimus dorsi at the sacrifice of decreasing the amount of scapular retraction that is performed. To isolate the muscles of the shoulder girdle and arms, avoid leaning backward while performing the exercise.

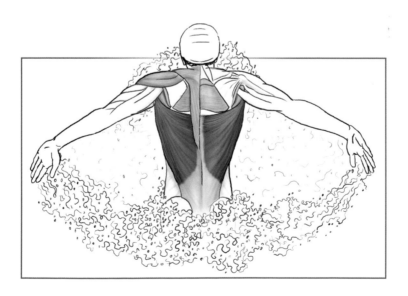

Bent-Over Single-Arm Row

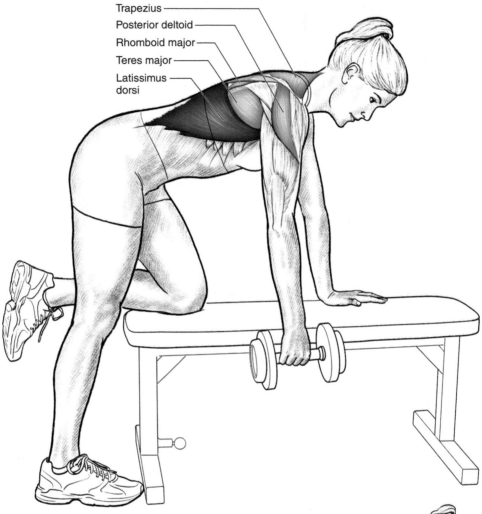

Trapezius
Posterior deltoid
Rhomboid major
Teres major
Latissimus dorsi

Execution

1. Holding a dumbbell in one hand, support your upper body with your free hand and knee on an exercise bench.

2. Keeping your spine straight, pull the dumbbell upward to your torso.

3. Raise your elbow as high as possible and pinch your shoulder blade back.

4. Slowly lower the weight to the starting position.

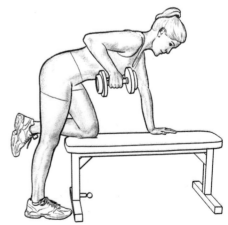

Finish position.

Muscles Involved

Primary: Latissimus dorsi

Secondary: Trapezius, rhomboid major, rhomboid minor, teres major, posterior deltoid, biceps brachii, brachialis

Swimming Focus

Similar to the seated row, this exercise is valuable for the breaststroker who wants to strengthen the second half of the pull. It is also a good general strengthening exercise that any swimmer can use to develop the strength of the latissimus dorsi.

When performing the exercise with a lighter weight, more emphasis is placed on the scapular retracting muscles. Using greater weight shifts the focus to the latissimus dorsi. Head positioning during this exercise is important. As with swimming, looking upward drops the hips and arches the low back, whereas looking downward toward the feet rolls the shoulders forward. To maintain the correct positioning, focus on a spot on the floor that is in line with the hand that is bracing your upper body. To help protect your low back, set your core muscles while performing this exercise. Doing this helps prevent excessive rotation of your upper body, which is a form of cheating.

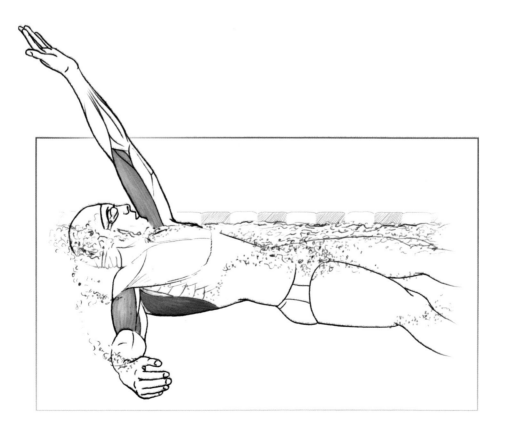

Standing Zeus

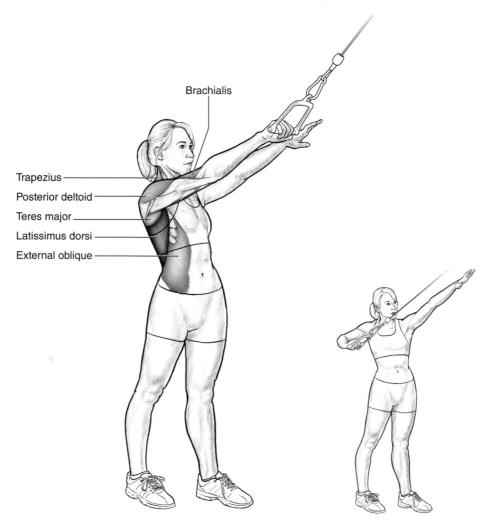

Brachialis

Trapezius

Posterior deltoid

Teres major

Latissimus dorsi

External oblique

Finish position.

Execution

1. Stand sideways to the pulley. Begin with both hands pointing upward at the pulley, although only one hand will be grasping the stirrup handle.

2. Keeping one hand stationary, pull the handle toward your upper chest while simultaneously rotating your chest backward.

3. In the ending position, emphasize pinching your shoulder blade backward.

4. Return to the starting position.

Muscles Involved

Primary: Latissimus dorsi

Secondary: Trapezius, rhomboid major, rhomboid minor, teres major, posterior deltoid, biceps brachii, brachialis, external oblique, internal oblique

Swimming Focus

This exercise ties movements of the shoulder girdle and arms to those of the trunk, in the process linking the recruitment of the latissimus dorsi to the internal and external obliques. This in turn strengthens the linkage between the arms and legs during freestyle and backstroke.

To emphasize the linkage between the core trunk musculature and the latissimus dorsi, focus on setting the core as described in the introduction to chapter 5. While performing the exercise, focus on keeping the elbow high throughout the entire range of motion.

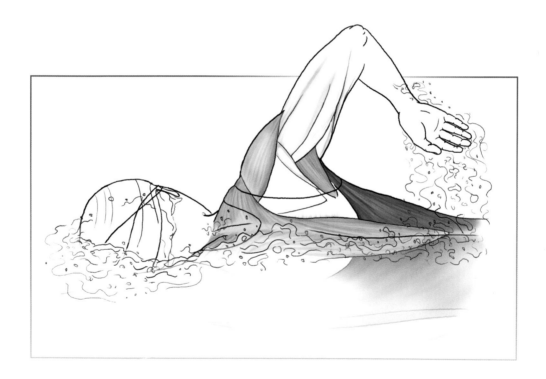

Lumbar Extension

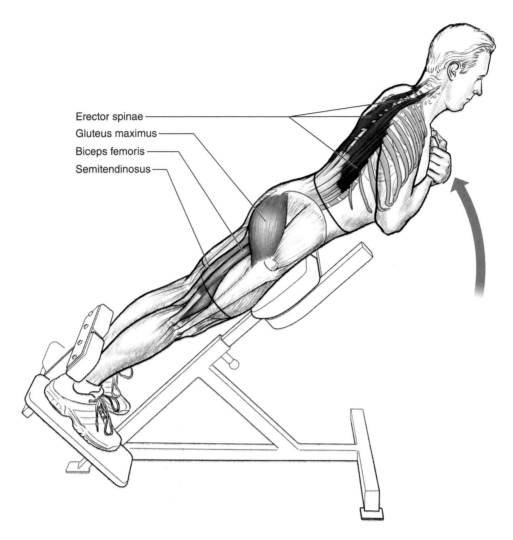

Erector spinae
Gluteus maximus
Biceps femoris
Semitendinosus

Execution

1. Lie facedown, position the bolster just below your hips, and secure your ankles.
2. From a hanging position, raise your torso until your legs and upper body are in a straight line.
3. Slowly lower your upper body back to the hanging position.

Muscles Involved

Primary: Erector spinae

Secondary: Gluteus maximus, biceps femoris, semitendinosus, semimembranosus

Swimming Focus

This exercise targets the primary and secondary muscles in a manner that is beneficial to several demands encountered while swimming the four competitive strokes. Butterfly and breaststroke swimmers will benefit through strengthening of the undulating or wavelike body movements that are integral to their movement through the water. The exercise also helps to strengthen the underwater dolphin kick. The exercise can also improve the start by helping the swimmer extend into a streamlined position off the blocks or, in the case of backstroke, by helping the swimmer get off the wall and into the water.

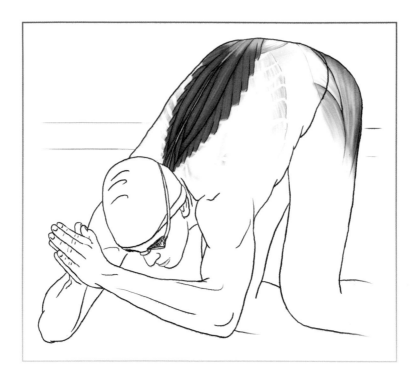

⚠ **SAFETY TIP** A slight degree of hyperextension, equal to the amount performed during butterfly or breaststroke recovery, is allowable, but amounts beyond that are discouraged to minimize the risk of injury.

VARIATION

Lumbar Extension With Rotation

A rotational component can be added to the ending position to mimic the long-axis rotation that the trunk undergoes during freestyle and backstroke swimming. Be careful to avoid hyperextending your back in the process of adding in the rotation component.

Physioball Back Extension

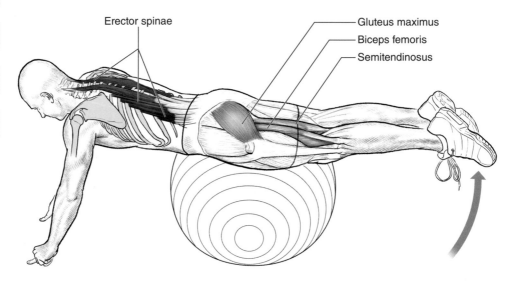

Erector spinae

Gluteus maximus
Biceps femoris
Semitendinosus

Execution

1. Begin facedown with a physioball positioned under your hips. Stabilize your upper body by resting your hands on the ground. Your legs should be straight, with just your toes touching the ground.
2. Lift your heels and shoulders upward, taking care not to extend your neck.
3. Pause at the top of the movement, using only your fingertips for balance.
4. Slowly return to the starting position.

Muscles Involved

Primary: Erector spinae

Secondary: Gluteus maximus, biceps femoris, semitendinosus, semimembranosus

Swimming Focus

The motions performed during this exercise closely mimic the undulating and wavelike body movements performed during butterfly, breaststroke, and underwater dolphin kicking. Although the exercise recruits the same muscles as the lumbar extension exercise, the range of motion performed is more limited, decreasing its benefit to enhancing starts. While performing the exercise, keeping the cervical spine and head in line with the rest of the spine is important in maintaining proper positioning of the lumbar and thoracic spine.

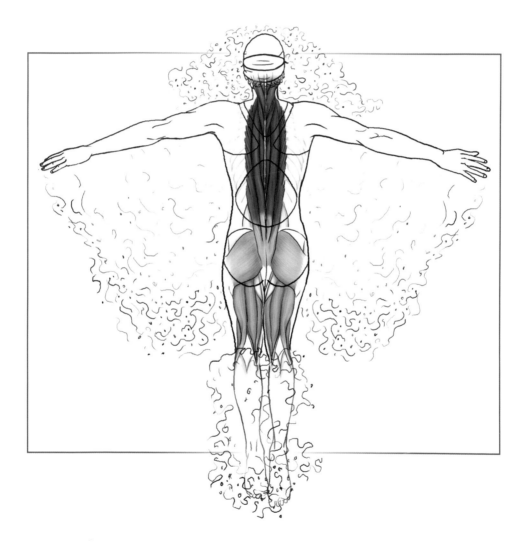

⚠ **SAFETY TIP** A slight degree of hyperextension, equal to the amount performed during butterfly or breaststroke recovery, is allowable, but amounts beyond that are discouraged to minimize the risk of injury.

Physioball Prone Superman Progression

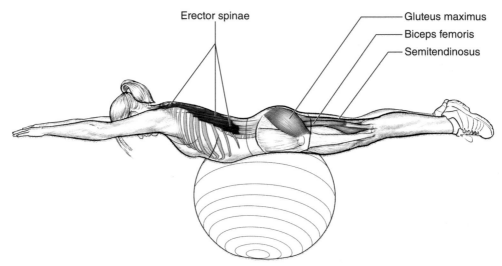

Execution

1. Begin facedown with a physioball positioned under your hips.
2. Lift your heels and shoulders upward, taking care not to extend your neck.
3. Move one arm to the streamlined position and use the other for balance.
4. Move the second arm to the streamlined position.
5. Hold this body position tightly for two to four seconds.
6. Reverse the movements.

Muscles Involved

Primary: Erector spinae

Secondary: Gluteus maximus, biceps femoris, semitendinosus, semimembranosus

Swimming Focus

Although this looks like a straightforward exercise, it is challenging to perform because it depends not necessarily on strength but on the ability to react dynamically to the challenge of balancing on the physioball while simultaneously holding the streamlined body position. Balance can be improved by first becoming comfortable with the physioball back extension exercise previously described. To transition into performing the full streamline, begin by alternating a single arm into the streamlined position while using the other hand for balance. You will find the exercise easier to perform by focusing first on positioning the legs and then slowly bringing the arms into position, rather than trying to get into position quickly. Slightly deflating the physioball will also make the exercise easier to perform.

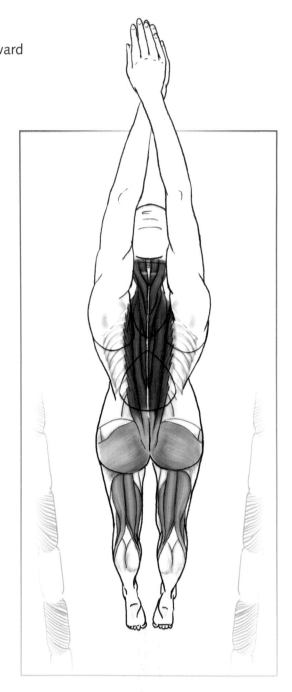

Physioball Prone Streamline

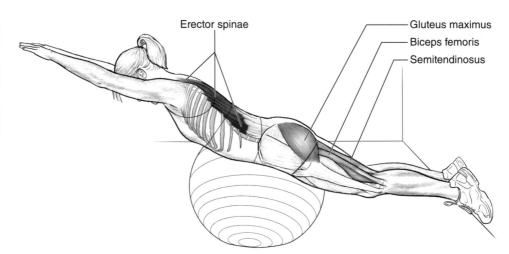

Erector spinae

Gluteus maximus

Biceps femoris

Semitendinosus

Execution

1. Begin with a physioball positioned under your abdomen. Brace your feet against a wall.
2. Push with your legs, rolling out over the ball until your body is in a straight line from your heels to the tip of your head.
3. As you extended your body forward, bring the arms into a streamlined position.
4. Slowly return to the starting position.

Muscles Involved

Primary: Erector spinae

Secondary: Gluteus maximus, biceps femoris, semitendinosus, semimembranosus

Swimming Focus

The goal of this exercise is to develop strength and confidence in holding a streamlined position. An advantage of this exercise is that on land, unlike in the water, a swimmer can be directly provided with feedback while holding the streamlined position.

A good place to start is the intermediate position, in which the arms are held along the sides instead of overhead as in a streamline. The transition from the intermediate to the advanced position can be progressed by reaching out with one arm at a time. The difficulty of the exercise can be varied by altering the positioning of the physioball. Positioning the ball closer to the feet increases the difficulty of the exercise, and moving it closer to the head makes the exercise easier.

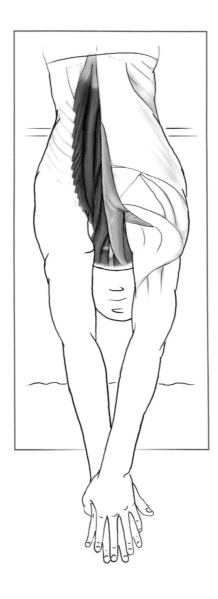

Physioball Bridge

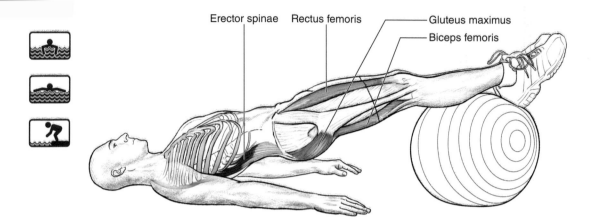

Erector spinae   Rectus femoris   Gluteus maximus   Biceps femoris

Execution

1. Lie on your back and position a physioball under your calves.
2. Tighten your core muscles and lift your hips toward the ceiling.
3. Hold your body in a straight line from your ankles to your shoulders.
4. Slowly lower back to the starting position.

Muscles Involved

Primary: Erector spinae

Secondary: Gluteus maximus, rectus femoris, biceps femoris, semitendinosus, semimembranosus

Swimming Focus

This exercise does an excellent job of tying activation of the gluteal and hamstring muscles to the core. Although you are facing upward when performing this exercise, it will strengthen the muscles that contribute to the undulating body movements that are performed during butterfly, breaststroke, and dolphin kicking.

Before raising your hips off the ground, set your core as described in chapter 5. Doing this will isolate the exercise to the primary and secondary muscle groups and prevent injury to the low back. The difficulty of the exercise can be varied by altering the position of your feet on the ball. The less contact you have with the ball, the more difficult the exercise will be. The highest level of difficulty occurs when only your heels are touching the top of the ball. This exercise also serves as the foundation for the physioball hamstring curl described in chapter 7.

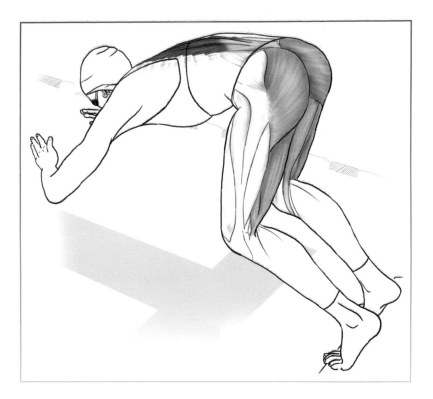

⚠️ **SAFETY TIP** Make sure that you maintain shoulder contact with the ground. You should not feel pressure on the head or neck when performing this exercise.

VARIATION

Single-Leg Physioball Bridge

This advanced version of the exercise should be initiated after you are able to maintain good control of your hips while performing the bridge exercise. The ultimate goal is to hold the hips in the bridged position, lift one leg for 5 seconds, lower it back to the ball, lift the opposite leg for 5 seconds, and then continue this alteration for 60 seconds.

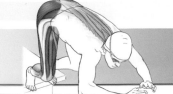
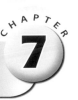
Strong legs are a critical component to reaching your true potential as a swimmer. They are not only the basis for having a powerful and efficient kick but also the key to driving your body off the starting blocks and turn walls. They also play an often overlooked role as a member of the kinetic chain by balancing your stroke mechanics and contributing to a tight streamline.

The lower extremity consists of three major joints—the hip, the knee, and the ankle. Five bones make up the three joints. The pelvis serves as the link between both legs and the torso. Each thigh is composed of a single long bone called the femur. The lower leg contains the tibia and fibula. The talus is the bone that serves as the connecting point between the ankle and lower leg. The hip joint is formed by the bony socket of the pelvis, called the acetabulum, and the head of the femur, which is shaped like a ball. The knee is the junction of the femur and the tibia, and the ankle is composed of the lower ends of the tibia and fibula and the upper part of the talus.

As a ball-and-socket joint, the hip is capable of a wide range of movements that can be described in three pairs. Flexion involves lifting the thigh upward toward the ceiling as if you are lifting your leg to climb a set of stairs. Extension is movement of the thigh backward. Abduction occurs when the leg is moved to the side away from the midline of the body, and adduction is the movement of bringing the leg back toward the midline of the body. Internal rotation is the process of touching the big toe of each foot together along the midline of the body. External rotation is the opposite and allows you to touch the back end of both heels together.

At the knee, a hinge joint, two primary movements occur. Flexion is the process of pulling the heel to the buttocks, and extension is straightening the knee from a flexed position. Four movements take place at the ankle joint. The process of pointing your toes, as you do in a tight streamline, is plantarflexion. Lifting your toes off the ground and toward your shin is called dorsiflexion. Rolling your ankle inward so that the bottom of your foot faces the midline of your body is inversion. Finally, eversion involves twisting your foot outward as you would before initiating a breaststroke kick.

The muscles of the leg can be categorized as those that act on the hip and knee and those that act on the ankle. The thigh and hip muscles can further be categorized into the following groupings: anterior, medial, gluteal, and posterior. Within the anterior grouping are seven muscles. The iliopsoas (figure 7.1 on page 142) is a deep muscle that arises from the anterior aspect of the lumbar vertebrae and the inner aspect of the pelvis and then crosses the hip joint to attach to the proximal femur. The primary movement generated by the iliopsoas is hip flexion. The quadriceps femoris, the largest muscle group in the body, is divided into four separate muscles that are named according to their point of origin. The rectus femoris, the only one to cross both the hip and knee, originates from the anterior aspect of the pelvis. The vastus lateralis arises from the lateral aspect of the femur, the vastus medialis arises from the medial aspect of the femur, and the vastus intermedius is in the middle. All four muscles have a common insertion on the anterior aspect of the tibia through the patellar tendon and function to extend the knee. Because the rectus femoris crosses the hip joint, it also functions as a hip flexor. The tensor fasciae latae (TFL) runs from the anterior aspect of the pelvis to combine with the iliotibial band (IT band), a thickened band of fascial tissue that runs down the lateral thigh. It then inserts on the lateral aspect of the tibia just below the knee joint. The primary actions of the TFL are hip flexion, abduction, and internal rotation. The final muscle of the anterior group is the sartorius, which is a long straplike muscle that runs diagonally from the anterior pelvis to the medial aspect of the tibia. Its primary actions are to flex, abduct, and externally rotate the hip.

The medial grouping can be divided into the adductor muscle family and two additional muscles that lie in close proximity. The adductor family is composed of three muscles (adductor magnus, adductor longus, and adductor brevis), which all arise from the inferior portion of the pelvis near the midline of the body and attach to the medial aspect of the femur. As the name implies, the primary function of

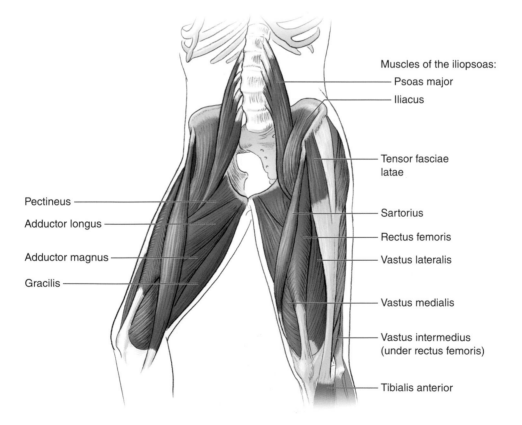

Figure 7.1   Muscles of the front of the legs.

this muscle family is hip adduction. Just superior to the adductors is the pectineus, which also originates from the inferior pelvis near the midline of the body and then inserts along the medial aspect of the femur. Besides assisting the adductors, the pectineus also flexes the hip. The gracilis is the most medial and inferior. It has the same origin as the other muscles but crosses the knee to attach on the medial aspect of the tibia just below the knee joint. Besides adducting the hip, the gracilis is also a secondary flexor of the knee.

The gluteal group contains the three gluteal muscles and a collection of six deep rotators. The gluteus maximus (figure 7.2), the largest and most superficial of the gluteal muscles, arises from the posterior half of the pelvis and a portion of an adjacent bone called the sacrum. It then crosses the hip joint to combine with the IT band, also attaching to a small portion of the femur. The main action of the gluteus maximus is extension of the hip. It also assists other muscles in the region with external rotation of the hip. The gluteus medius and minimus both lie deep to the gluteus maximus and arise from the lateral part of the pelvis. The two muscles cross the hip joint, attaching to a bony prominence on the femur called the greater trochanter. Both muscles function to abduct and internally rotate the hip. The deep rotators are a collection of six small muscles (piriformis, gemellus superior, gemellus inferior, obturator externus, obturator internus, and quadratus femoris) that combine to rotate the hip externally and, like the rotator cuff at the shoulder, stabilize the hip joint.

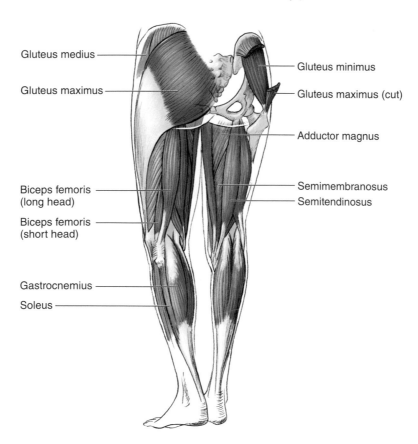

Figure 7.2 Muscles of the back of the legs.

The posterior group is composed of the three hamstring muscles. The biceps femoris, as the name implies, has two heads, one arising from a part of the pelvis called the ischial tuberosity and the other arising from the lower posterior aspect of the femur. The two heads combine to form a common tendon that inserts on the head of the fibula. The other two hamstring muscles, the semitendinosus and semimembranosus, also originate from the ischial tuberosity but run along the medial aspect of the knee joint to attach at the medial surface of the superior part of the tibia. Collectively, the muscles extend the hip and flex the knee.

The muscles of the lower leg can be grouped according to their actions at the ankle joint. The gastrocnemius and soleus are the primary plantarflexors and share an insertion into the Achilles tendon. The tibialis anterior and posterior, named according to their attachment location on the tibia, function to invert the foot. The fibularis muscle group (fibularis tertius, fibularis brevis, and fibularis longus), located on the lateral aspect of the ankle joint, originates from the fibula and has the primary function of foot eversion.

For discussion purposes, the muscle recruitment patterns of the freestyle and backstroke flutter kick are described jointly because the patterns are practically identical. The propulsive portion of the flutter kick begins with the torso and core-stabilizing musculature acting as the foundation on which your legs generate their force. The actual kicking movements begin with the hips in a small amount of extension. From this extended position the iliopsoas and rectus femoris are activated to initiate hip flexion. Also acting on the knee joint, the rectus femoris initiates knee extension and is quickly joined by the remainder of the quadriceps group, which helps to increase the force produced during the kick. These muscles remain active throughout the entire propulsive phase of the kick. At the ankle joint, the tibialis anterior and tibialis posterior work in concert to maintain the foot in a position of slight inversion, while contraction of the gastrocnemius and soleus plantarflexes the foot. The hip extension that takes place during the recovery phase is guided by the hamstrings and gluteus maximus. Unlike in flutter kicking, during butterfly and dolphin kicking the torso serves not only as the foundation for the kick but also as a component. The undulating body movements of the torso initiate the kick, and paired movements of the legs follow in a manner identical to the action of the flutter kick. One difference in the paired movement of the legs is that a greater amount of flexion and extension occurs at both the hips and knees. The undulating movement of the torso is guided by the contraction of the abdominal and erector spinae muscles, but the muscles that guide the movements of the legs are identical to those used in the flutter kick.

The starting point for the propulsive phase of the breaststroke kick is with the feet 8 to 10 inches (20 to 25 cm) apart and the knees and hips flexed. From this position the TFL, gluteus medius, and gluteus minimus internally rotate and abduct the hips, which results in the legs further separating from each other. As the ankles begin to separate, the biceps femoris contracts, pulling on the outer portion of the lower leg, which externally rotates the lower leg and results in further separation of the ankles. At the same time the fibularis muscle group contracts to evert the foot. These combined movements place the legs in the position to begin the whip portion of the kick. From this position the gluteus maximus contracts forcefully to extend the hip, the quadriceps muscle group functions to extend the knee, and the powerful adductor muscles (adductor magnus, adductor longus, adductor brevis, pectineus, and gracilis) pull both legs back toward the midline of the body. At the ankle joint the tibialis posterior, gastrocnemius, and soleus contract to return the ankle to a streamlined plantarflexed position for the glide portion of the stroke. Recovery is accomplished by recruitment of the rectus femoris and iliopsoas, which serve to flex the hip, and recruitment of the hamstrings, which serve to flex the knee.

Back Squat

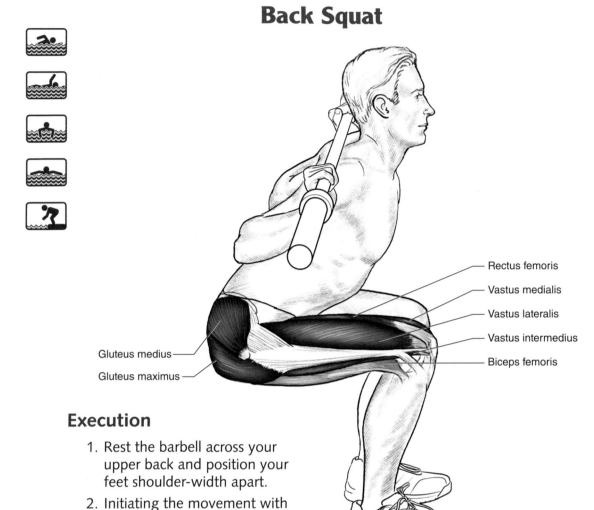

Rectus femoris
Vastus medialis
Vastus lateralis
Vastus intermedius
Biceps femoris

Gluteus medius
Gluteus maximus

Execution

1. Rest the barbell across your upper back and position your feet shoulder-width apart.
2. Initiating the movement with your hips, squat down until your thighs are parallel to the ground.
3. Return to the starting position by straightening your legs.

Muscles Involved

Primary: Rectus femoris, vastus medialis, vastus intermedius, vastus lateralis, gluteus maximus, gluteus medius

Secondary: Erector spinae, biceps femoris, semitendinosus, semimembranosus, adductor magnus, adductor longus, adductor brevis, pectineus, sartorius, gracilis, transversus abdominis, external oblique, internal oblique

⚠️ **SAFETY TIP** Improper squat technique is one of the leading causes of injuries during dryland or weight-room training. Be sure to start with a light weight and add weight only when you have become comfortable with performing the lift and have had a certified strength and conditioning professional review your technique.

Swimming Focus

Squats are a good all-around exercise because they recruit all major muscles groups of the lower extremity. Increasing the strength of the knee extensors transfers to improved force generation and endurance when kicking, regardless of stroke. Strengthening of the gluteal muscles, specifically the gluteus maximus, helps to improve the force that is generated with the extension of the hip during the breaststroke kick. Because of the similarities in the movements performed in squats and starts, particularly

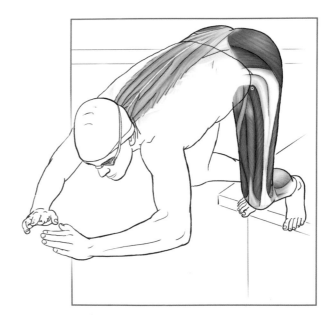

flat starts, squats should be a mainstay exercise for enhancing a swimmer's start.

Extra caution should be used because of the potential for injury to the low back or knees. To protect the low back, beginners should start with just the bar until they are fully comfortable with the exercise. Emphasizing tightening of the core musculature, as described in the introduction to chapter 5, will also help protect the low back. The most common causes for injury to the knee are shifting of the knees forward past the toes or allowing the knees to collapse inward when squatting down.

VARIATION

Overhead Squat

Advantages of overhead squats are that they place a focus on maintaining an upright body posture and develop strength and confidence with the arms in an overhead position. Weight used is much less than in a traditional squat, so starting this exercise with a wooden dowel is best.

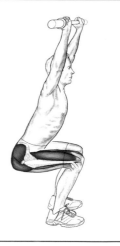

Single-Leg Squat

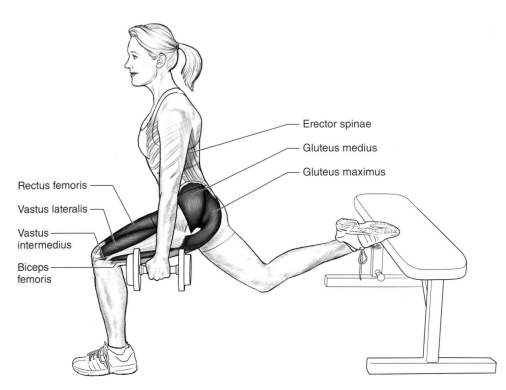

Erector spinae

Gluteus medius

Gluteus maximus

Rectus femoris

Vastus lateralis

Vastus intermedius

Biceps femoris

Execution

1. With a dumbbell in each hand, stand 2 feet (60 cm) in front of a flat bench and position your feet hip-width apart.
2. Reach back with one foot and rest your toes on the bench.
3. Initiating the movement with your hips, lower your body until the thigh of the standing leg is near parallel to the ground.
4. Return to the starting position by straightening your leg.

Muscles Involved

Primary: Rectus femoris, vastus medialis, vastus intermedius, vastus lateralis, gluteus maximus, gluteus medius

Secondary: Erector spinae, biceps femoris, semitendinosus, semimembranosus, adductor magnus, adductor longus, adductor brevis, pectineus, sartorius, gracilis, transversus abdominis, external oblique, internal oblique

Swimming Focus

Like double-leg squats, single-leg squats target all the major muscle groups of the lower extremity. An advantage of single-leg squats is that they isolate one leg at a time, which can help address muscle imbalances that may exist between the legs. Targeting all the major muscle groups of the lower extremity improves kicking strength and endurance as well as strength with starts and turns.

During the exercise, you should use the back leg for balance purposes only. As your confidence and balance improve, you can substitute a physioball for a bench. Give extra attention to the positioning of your knee as you lower into the squatting position. Repeated inward dropping of the knee and forward translation past the toes are technique flaws. If you notice these flaws, modify either the weight or number of repetitions to reduce the intensity of the exercise.

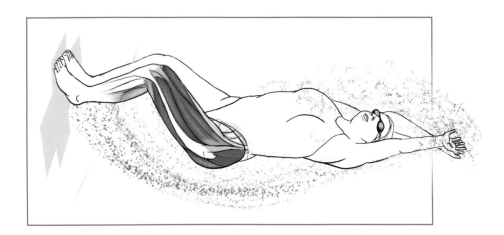

Dumbbell Step-Up

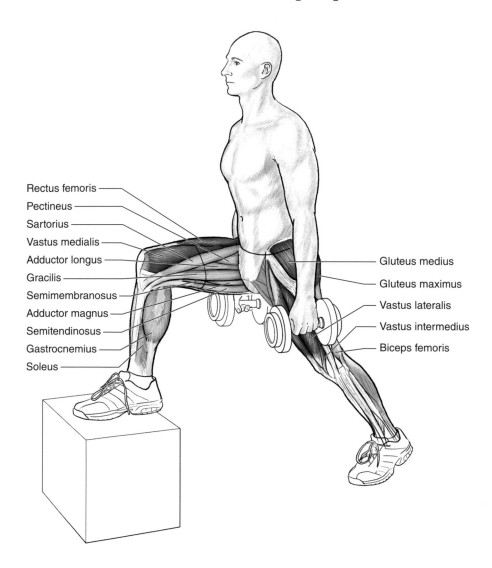

Rectus femoris
Pectineus
Sartorius
Vastus medialis
Adductor longus
Gracilis
Semimembranosus
Adductor magnus
Semitendinosus
Gastrocnemius
Soleus

Gluteus medius
Gluteus maximus
Vastus lateralis
Vastus intermedius
Biceps femoris

Execution

1. Holding a dumbbell in each hand, stand facing a box.
2. Step up onto the box with one leg. Pressing through this leg, lift yourself upward until both feet are on the box.
3. Step down with the leg that initiated the exercise.
4. Repeat, initiating the exercise with the opposite leg.

⚠ **SAFETY TIP** To protect the low back, you must maintain a tall, upright posture during the entire exercise. A common technique flaw is leaning the upper trunk forward.

Muscles Involved

Primary: Rectus femoris, vastus medialis, vastus intermedius, vastus lateralis, psoas major, gluteus maximus, gluteus medius

Secondary: Biceps femoris, semitendinosus, semimembranosus, adductor magnus, adductor longus, adductor brevis, pectineus, sartorius, gracilis, gastrocnemius, soleus, transversus abdominis, external oblique, internal oblique

Swimming Focus

Dumbbell step-ups are another good exercise for targeting all the major muscle groups of the lower extremity at the same time. Strength gains will carry over to improved strength and distance off the starting blocks, especially with track starts because of the single-leg isolation, as well as turn walls. Targeting of the knee extensors will transfer to force development and stamina with kicking.

To maximize the benefit of the exercise, emphasize a slow, controlled descent from the top of the box. The difficulty of the exercise can be modified by altering the height of the box.

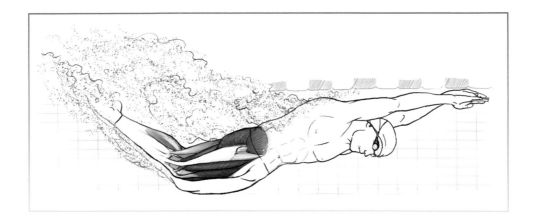

VARIATION

Barbell Step-Up

As your strength improves, using dumbbells may become impractical, at which time you can implement the use of a barbell. When using a barbell, rest it on the trapezius as if you were performing a barbell squat, but be aware that the weight will shift farther from the center of gravity compared with using dumbbells. Be ready for a change in balance.

Lunge

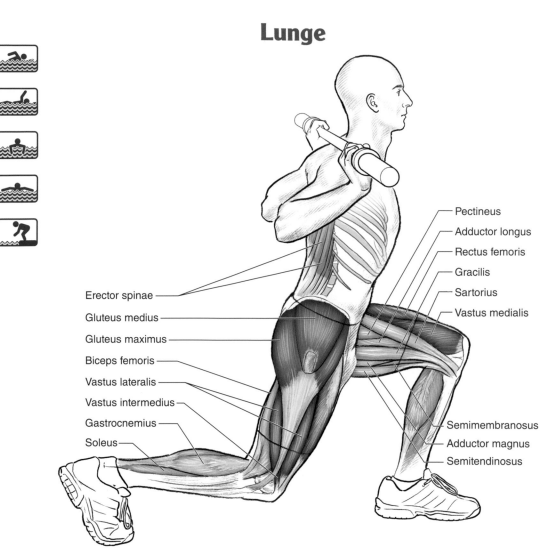

Erector spinae
Gluteus medius
Gluteus maximus
Biceps femoris
Vastus lateralis
Vastus intermedius
Gastrocnemius
Soleus

Pectineus
Adductor longus
Rectus femoris
Gracilis
Sartorius
Vastus medialis

Semimembranosus
Adductor magnus
Semitendinosus

Execution

1. Rest the barbell across your upper back and position your feet shoulder-width apart.
2. Step forward, bending the knee of your front leg until your thigh is parallel to the ground. Avoid allowing the back knee to touch the ground.
3. Push back with the front foot to return to the starting position.

Muscles Involved

Primary: Rectus femoris, vastus medialis, vastus intermedius, vastus lateralis, gluteus maximus, gluteus medius

Secondary: Erector spinae, biceps femoris, semitendinosus, semimembranosus, adductor magnus, adductor longus, adductor brevis, pectineus, sartorius, gracilis, gastrocnemius, soleus, transversus abdominis, external oblique, internal oblique

Swimming Focus

This exercise engages all the major muscle groups of the lower extremity in a dynamic fashion that incorporates a balance component. Use of this exercise will lead to improved kicking performance and have a beneficial effect on starts and turns.

To avoid leaning your torso forward during the exercise, in the starting position pick an object at eye level and maintain focus on that object throughout the entire lunge. By using this technique your head will stay up, and subsequently your torso will remain upright. Pay close attention to the position of your knee in relation to your foot. In the ending position your lower leg should be perpendicular to the ground.

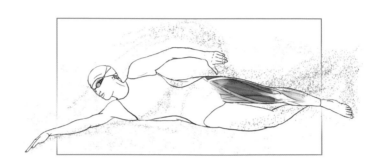

VARIATIONS

Walking Lunge

To perform this variation, instead of pushing back, shift your weight forward. Push off your front leg and bring your back leg to the forward position, recreating the lunge position.

Diagonal and Lateral Lunge

The diagonal and lateral movements increase the demands placed on the adductor muscle group, which will be of extra benefit to breaststrokers. To mix up a dryland program, try replacing forward lunges with a repeating cycle of a forward lunge followed by a diagonal lunge and then a lateral lunge.

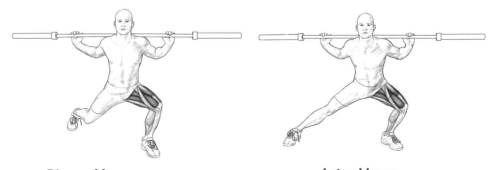

Diagonal lunge.   Lateral lunge.

Standing Hip Internal Rotation

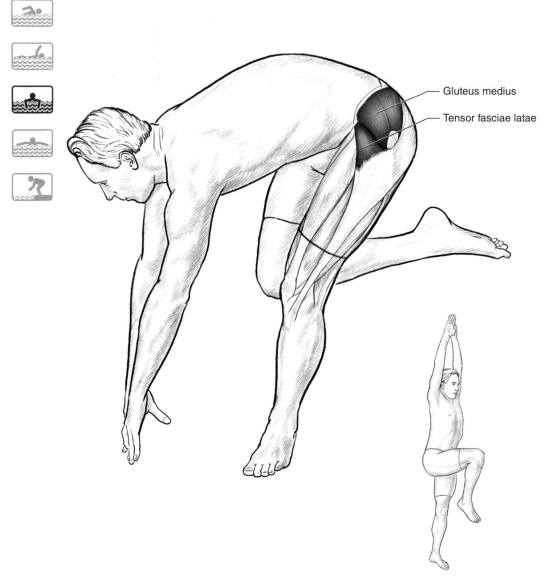

Gluteus medius

Tensor fasciae latae

Finish position.

Execution

1. Standing on one leg, reach with your arms and trunk to the inner side of the weight-bearing foot.
2. Use the weight-bearing leg as a pivot point.
3. Reach your arms and trunk toward a point on the ceiling above and slightly behind the same shoulder.
4. Hold the free leg in a flexed position and simultaneously rotate it with the trunk, driving the knee upward toward the ceiling with the arms.

Muscles Involved

Primary: Tensor fasciae latae, gluteus medius, gluteus minimus

Secondary: None

Swimming Focus

This exercise targets a select group of muscles that are responsible for internal rotation of the hips, a movement that is primarily seen in swimming during the recovery phase of the breaststroke kick as the heels are brought toward the buttocks. Breaststrokers will therefore benefit most from the exercise. But other swimmers should not ignore the exercise, because a small rotational component takes place during the other strokes. Like the rotator cuff muscles of the shoulder, these muscles play a protective role and help stabilize the hip joint. This exercise is also useful for teaching balance and postural control, especially for younger swimmers.

Emphasis should be placed on the rotational movements performed during exercise because this is the key to targeting the rotary muscles. The knee extensors and gluteus maximus can also be incorporated by adding a slight knee bend as you reach toward the ground. As your confidence and strength grow, you can hold a medicine ball in both hands to increase the difficulty of the exercise.

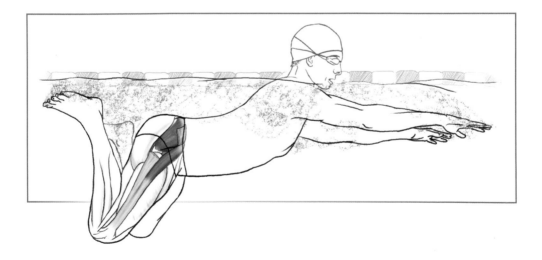

Standing Hip External Rotation

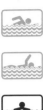

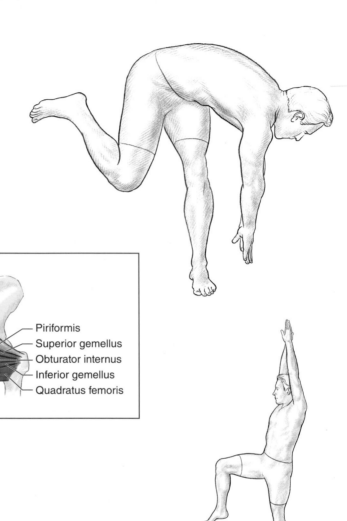

Piriformis
Superior gemellus
Obturator internus
Inferior gemellus
Quadratus femoris
Obturator externus

Finish position.

Execution

1. Standing on one leg, reach with your arms and trunk to the outer side of the weight-bearing foot.
2. Use the weight-bearing leg as a pivot point.
3. Reach your arms and trunk toward a point on the ceiling above and slightly behind the opposite shoulder.
4. Hold the free leg in a flexed position and simultaneously rotate it with the trunk, driving the knee upward toward the ceiling with the arms.

Muscles Involved

Primary: Obturator internus, superior gemellus, inferior gemellus, obturator externus, quadratus femoris

Secondary: Piriformis, gluteus maximus, sartorius

Swimming Focus

By targeting a group of muscles that are responsible for externally rotating the hip, this exercise can help increase the forces generated during the propulsive phase of the breaststroke kick. Like the hip's internal rotators, the external rotators also function as hip stabilizers, making this an exercise that all swimmers should consider for injury prevention purposes. The single-leg nature of the exercise and combined movements of the upper trunk also make this a useful exercise for improving balance and linking movements between the upper and lower extremities. As mentioned in the previous exercise, the emphasis should be on maintaining balance and the rotational movements. The knee extensors and gluteus maximus can also be incorporated by adding a slight knee bend as you reach toward the ground. As your confidence and strength grow, you can hold a medicine ball in both hands to increase the difficulty of the exercise.

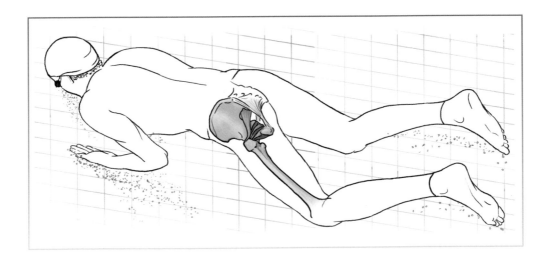

Romanian Deadlifts (RDLs)

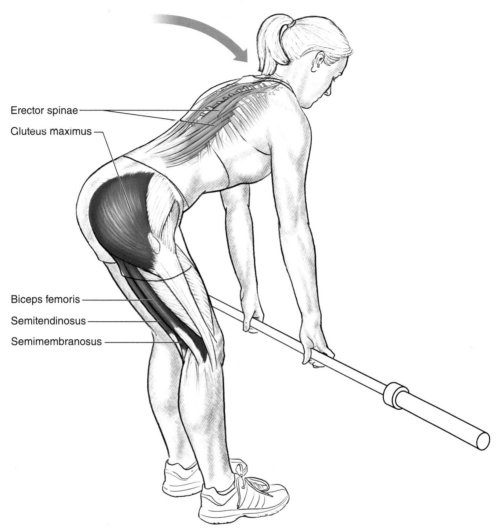

Erector spinae

Gluteus maximus

Biceps femoris

Semitendinosus

Semimembranosus

Execution

1. Holding a barbell with an overhand grip, position your feet shoulder-width apart.
2. Bend your knees slightly.
3. Keeping your back straight, start lowering the bar by pushing your hips backward.
4. Lower the bar until you feel a stretch in your hamstrings.
5. Rise back up to the starting position.

Muscles Involved

Primary: Gluteus maximus, biceps femoris, semitendinosus, semimembranosus

Secondary: Erector spinae

Swimming Focus

The primary targets of RDLs are the gluteus maximus and the hamstring muscle group, muscles that are important in extending the hips when performing starts and when transitioning into a streamlined position off each turn wall. The gluteal muscles and hamstrings are also important in extending the hips during the propulsive portion of the breaststroke kick.

To ensure proper performance of the exercise, focus on the following: (1) Keep your head up because looking downward will roll the shoulders and place extra stress on the back, (2) keep the back flat during the entire movement, and (3) isolate the movement to the hips.

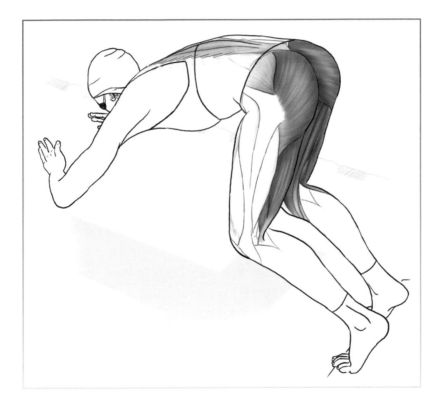

⚠ **SAFETY TIP** If performed improperly, especially when using heavier weights, this exercise presents a risk of injury, so younger swimmers should avoid it.

Physioball Hamstring Curl

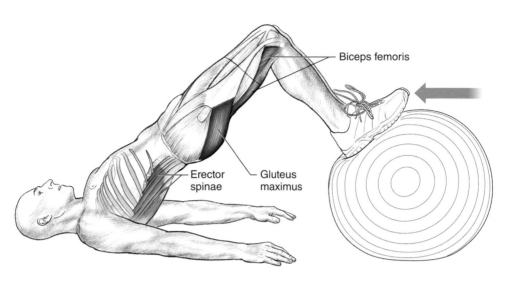

Biceps femoris

Erector spinae

Gluteus maximus

Execution

1. Lie on your back and position a physioball under your heels.
2. Tighten your core muscles and lift your hips toward the ceiling.
3. Without letting your hips drop, pull your heels toward your buttocks.
4. Straighten your legs until your body is in a straight line extending from your ankles to your shoulders. Then repeat.

Muscles Involved

Primary: Gluteus maximus, biceps femoris, semitendinosus, semimembranosus

Secondary: Erector spinae

Swimming Focus

Breaststrokers who want to strengthen their hamstrings will find this a useful exercise. This exercise is also valuable because it targets the hamstrings, gluteus maximus, and erector spinae, which contribute to holding a tight streamlined position. Those who do not have access to a formal weight room will find this a good exercise for the hamstrings because the only equipment needed is a physioball.

Before implementing this exercise, you must first master the physioball bridge exercise described in chapter 6 (page 138). To maintain proper body position, the core muscles must be activated during the entire exercise. Failure to recruit the core stabilizers will cause the hips to drop downward and decrease the effectiveness of the exercise. To avoid placing undue stress on the neck and head, make sure that you maintain shoulder contact with the ground.

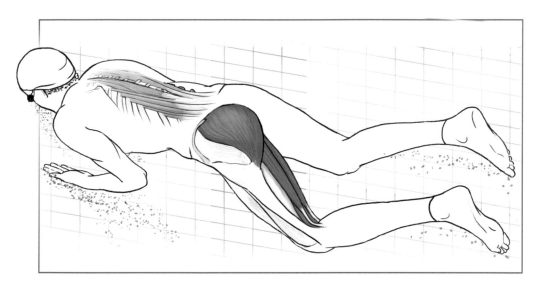

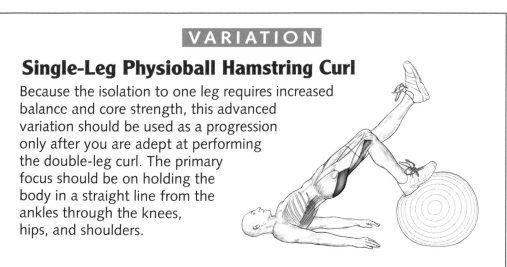

VARIATION

Single-Leg Physioball Hamstring Curl

Because the isolation to one leg requires increased balance and core strength, this advanced variation should be used as a progression only after you are adept at performing the double-leg curl. The primary focus should be on holding the body in a straight line from the ankles through the knees, hips, and shoulders.

Leg Curl

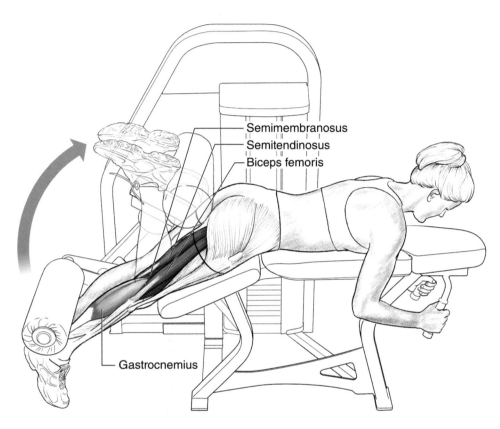

Semimembranosus
Semitendinosus
Biceps femoris

Gastrocnemius

Execution

1. Lie facedown on a hamstring curl machine and hook your heels under the roller pads.
2. Pull your heels toward your buttocks in an arcing motion.
3. Slowly lower the weight to the starting position.

Muscles Involved

Primary: Biceps femoris, semitendinosus, semimembranosus

Secondary: Gastrocnemius

Swimming Focus

Although the hamstrings actively contribute to the kicking motions performed during all four strokes, their involvement is greatest in the recovery phase of the breaststroke kick as the heels are drawn toward the buttocks. Swimmers tend to be quad dominant, resulting in a strength imbalance between the quadriceps and hamstrings. To address this imbalance, swimmers should incorporate exercises that isolate the hamstrings.

Breaststrokers should rotate the toes outward to mimic more closely the movements performed in the water. This positioning also increases recruitment of the biceps femoris. Avoid lifting the hips off the bench when performing the exercise. Perform the movements in a slow, controlled fashion. Do not try to kick the roller pads toward your buttocks; pull them instead.

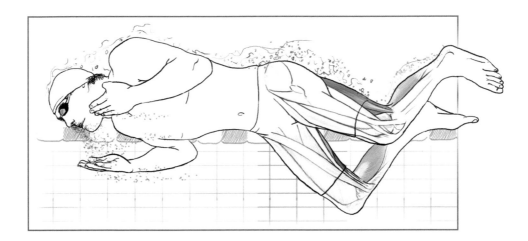

Leg Extension

Rectus femoris
Vastus lateralis
Vastus intermedius

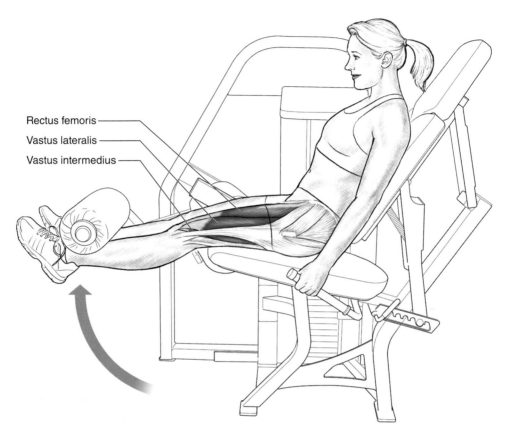

Execution

1. Sit on the leg extension machine and hook your ankles under the roller pads.
2. Extend your legs until your knees are straight.
3. Slowly lower your legs back down to the starting position.

Muscles Involved

Primary: Rectus femoris, vastus lateralis, vastus intermedius, vastus medialis

Secondary: None

Swimming Focus

This exercise directly targets the quadriceps muscle group and the rectus femoris in a manner that helps to strengthen the propulsive kicking phase of all four strokes. The same muscles also contribute to the lower-extremity movements that take place during starts and when pushing off a turn wall.

To maximize the benefit of the exercise, you must fully extend the knees in the ending position and lower the weight in a slow, controlled manner. When performing the exercise, focus on pushing the roller pads as opposed to trying to kick them toward the ceiling.

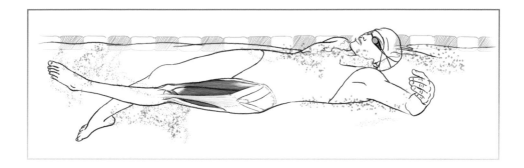

⚠ **SAFETY TIP** Swimmers who are currently experiencing knee pain or have a recent history of it should avoid this exercise because it can place increased stress on the patellar tendon and the undersurface of the patella (kneecap) as it glides over the femur.

Band Lateral Shuffle

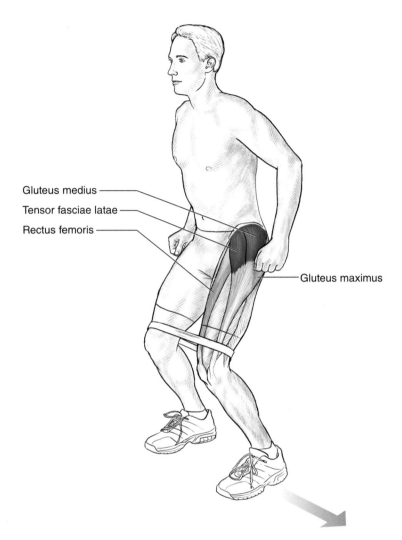

Gluteus medius
Tensor fasciae latae
Rectus femoris
Gluteus maximus

Execution

1. Stand with a slight bend in the knees and with the feet shoulder-width apart.
2. Keeping the trailing leg stationary, step to the side 12 to 18 inches (30 to 45 cm) with the lead leg.
3. After placing the lead foot on the ground, move the trailing foot.
4. Repeat steps 2 and 3 until you cover a set distance or number of repetitions.

Muscles Involved

Primary: Tensor fasciae latae, gluteus medius

Secondary: Gluteus maximus, rectus femoris

Swimming Focus

The tensor fasciae latae and gluteus medius are two important stabilizers of the pelvis. They also make minor contributions to the kicking movements that take place with all four strokes. Strengthening of these muscles is often overlooked in dryland programs. This exercise should be cycled into the dryland program at various times during the year to ensure that the muscles do not become neglected. Breaststrokers, who depend more on strong and stable hips, should incorporate it more often. The involvement of the rectus femoris and gluteus maximus can be increased by increasing the amount of knee flexion.

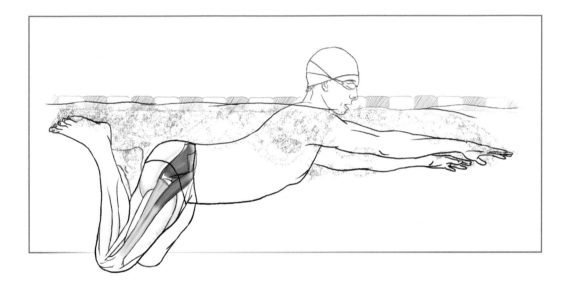

⚠️ **SAFETY TIP** Placing the exercise band below the knee can put undue stress on the tendons and ligaments surrounding the knee.

V A R I A T I O N

Band Diagonal Shuffle

Adding the diagonal movement will greatly increase the activation of the rectus femoris, which can improve kicking strength across all the strokes. This variation, however, will decrease the activation of the gluteus medius.

Standing Hip Adduction

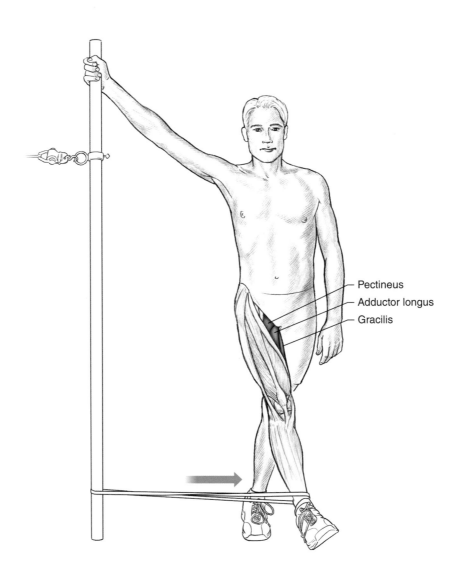

Pectineus
Adductor longus
Gracilis

Execution

1. Stand sideways to a backstroke flagpole with a band fixed to the pole and the ankle closer to the pole. Tighten your core muscles to stabilize your hips.
2. Allow the resistance of the band to pull your leg out to the side.
3. Keeping your knee straight, pull your leg across and in front of the stabilizing leg.
4. Slowly return to the starting position.

Muscles Involved

Primary: Adductor magnus, adductor longus, adductor brevis, pectineus, gracilis

Secondary: Transversus abdominis, external oblique, internal oblique

Swimming Focus

Direct targeting of the adductor muscle group can help the breaststroker increase the strength and stamina of the kick.

When performing the exercise, tightening the core stabilizers and holding the upper body in a tall, upright posture will help to isolate the adductor muscle group. Swimmers who are currently experiencing or have a recent history of knee pain should anchor the resistance band just above the knee.

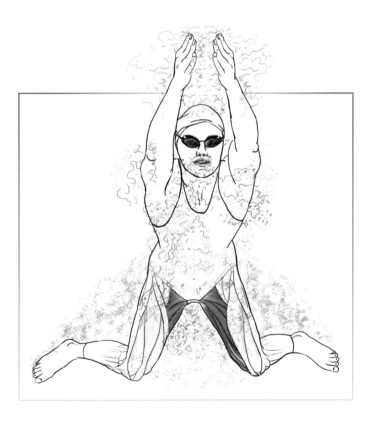

Inversion and Eversion Ankle Band Strengthening

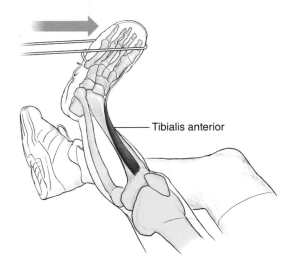

Tibialis anterior

Inversion.

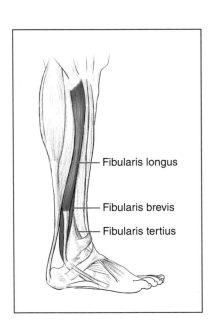

Fibularis longus

Fibularis brevis

Fibularis tertius

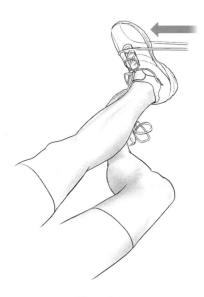

Eversion.

Execution for Inversion

1. Supporting the foot off the ground, wrap the exercise band around the forefoot so that the resistance is coming from an anchor point to the outside of the foot performing the exercise.

2. Without rotating the knee or hip, pull the toes toward the midline of the body.

3. Slowly return to the starting position.

Execution for Eversion

1. Supporting the foot off the ground, wrap the exercise band around the forefoot so that the resistance is coming from an anchor point to the inside of the foot performing the exercise.

2. Without rotating the knee or hip, pull the toes away from the midline of the body.

3. Slowly return to the starting position.

Muscles Involved

Primary: Tibialis anterior and tibialis posterior (invertors); fibularis longus and fibularis brevis (evertors)

Secondary: Flexor digitorum longus and flexor hallucis longus (invertors); fibularis tertius (evertor)

Swimming Focus

The ankle invertors (tibialis anterior and tibialis posterior) and the ankle evertors (fibularis muscle group) are important stabilizers of the ankle joint. Incorporation of exercises targeting these muscles can help protect the ankle joint by improving its dynamic stability. Strong ankle invertors provide support to the ankle during flutter and fly kicking and help maintain the foot in a slightly inverted position. Strengthening the ankle evertors helps with the positioning of the ankle and foot as the legs are being set for the whip portion of the breaststroke kick. The ankle evertors also provide lateral stability to the ankle, which can help protect against ankle sprains when performing cross-training activities such as running.

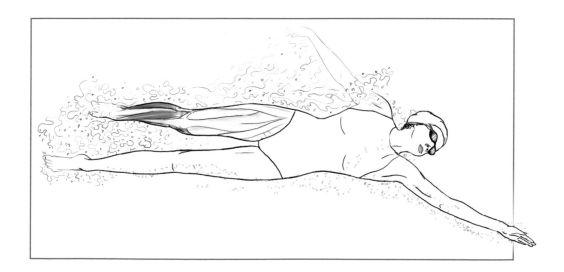

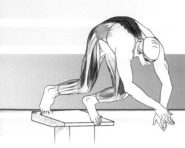

WHOLE-BODY TRAINING

This chapter focuses on whole-body exercises that require simultaneous muscle activation from muscles of the upper extremity, core, and lower extremity. Because the previous chapters discussed the specifics of joint and muscle anatomy, muscle actions, and their role in swimming, the focus of this chapter is to describe the importance of whole-body training and the role of these exercises in enhancing swimming performance.

The focus of the previous chapters has been on exercises that isolate a single joint or, through a combination of movements, the joints of the upper extremity or lower extremity. In contrast, the exercises in this chapter integrate the upper and lower extremities during total-body movements, allowing one exercise to link these areas with the core. These exercises involve multiple joints and multiple muscle groups and are therefore very functional, or sport specific.

As the number of joints and muscle groups recruited during an exercise increases, so does the specificity of the exercise. For example, a simple triceps extension isolates one joint, the elbow, and one muscle group, the triceps brachii. Comparatively, the burpee, an exercise described later in this chapter, is a total-body exercise that incorporates movements of the lower extremity and upper extremity and, in turn, multiple muscle groups. The differences between the two kinds of exercises are obvious; the question that arises concerns the comparative advantages and disadvantages of each. The primary advantage of the triceps extension is that it isolates a single muscle group. As a result, controlling the degree of resistance (by increasing or decreasing the weight) placed on the muscle is easy, and the focus can be directed to strengthening only the triceps. The main disadvantage is that the movement is not swimming specific because it involves only a single joint. On the other hand, the primary advantage of the burpee exercise is that multiple joints and muscle groups are involved and it emphasizes jumping into a streamline at the end of the exercise; it is a swimming-specific exercise. Other advantages are that it requires coordinated movements, activates the core musculature, and includes an explosive jumping component. Through the coordinated movements of the upper and lower extremities and activation of the core musculature, swimmers will find that these exercises help to improve the strength and efficiency of the strokes. A disadvantage of burpees and other total-body exercises is that because multiple muscle groups are recruited in unison, stronger muscles may compensate for weaker muscles. For example, an amazingly fast swimmer may also be the slowest kicker on the team if his or her upper-body stroke mechanics are strong enough to compensate for the lower-extremity kicking weakness. Although total-body exercises are important, you need to perform the more focused upper-body and lower-body multijoint movements and additional isolation exercises to have a comprehensive dryland program. Think of the total-body movements as your main set and the other exercises as the drills and technique work that fine-tune your stroke.

Besides having a total-body focus, several of the exercises emphasize explosive movements. The principle of specificity applies here. The best way to improve your ability to explode off the starting blocks and turn walls is to incorporate explosive exercises into the dryland program. The primary focus with these exercises is to help you learn to generate power through the lower extremity and core. The advantage of using exercise outside the pool to increase power production is that performing multiple repetitions in succession is easier, and technique feedback and corrections are more easily provided.

With these exercises come some special considerations. The first is that because these exercises incorporate multiple joint movements, the joint movements must be properly coordinated. An example of a poorly coordinated exercise would be to start the streamline before starting the jump when performing the burpee exercise. Initiating the streamline early removes the force-generating swinging motion of the arms that helps you jump higher. A swimming analogy would be to bring your arms into a streamlined position before initiating your jumping motion off the starting block. Lack of coordination can turn a total-body movement into several isolated single-joint exercises, decreasing the sport specificity. Additionally, because of the complicated nature of the exercises, technique perfection should be imperative. Therefore, when first using these exercises, you should focus on the quality of the movement, not the quantity. This advice is especially relevant with the jumping and explosive exercises, not only because uncontrolled explosive movements present a high risk for injuries but also because the associated landings place increased stress on the lower extremities. One way to ensure proper technique is to begin these exercises by using little or no weight to engrain proper technique before building strength or power. A final consideration is the importance of the core-stabilizing musculature when performing these exercises. The core stabilizers function not only as the link between upper- and lower-body movements but also as stabilizers and protectors of the upper and lower back. Therefore, you must set the core stabilizers at the start of every exercise. Chapter 5 provides a thorough overview of how to set the core stabilizers.

A group of total-body exercises known as the Olympic lifts are extremely beneficial in developing speed, strength, and power. But because these complex exercises require teaching and supervision by qualified personnel (such as certified strength coaches), they are not included in this text. Two of the more common Olympic lifts that should be considered for advanced swimmers, when adequate instruction and supervision are available, are the hang clean and the hang snatch. These are two of the best total-body exercises for developing power through the core and lower extremity. Swimmers who specialize in the sprint events (50 to 100 meters or yards) will benefit the most from these lifts. The primary gains will be in explosiveness off the starting blocks and turn walls. Because of the skills required to perform these exercises, guidance should be obtained from a certified Olympic weightlifting coach or a certified strength and conditioning specialist.

All the exercises included in this chapter are beneficial because they are total-body in nature and, like the Olympic lifts, help to generate strength and power through the core. Advantages of these exercises are that they do not necessarily require instruction and supervision by a certified strength coach. As a general reminder, you should always have a coach supervise your program so that you can receive continual feedback on your technique.

Single-Arm Lawn Mower

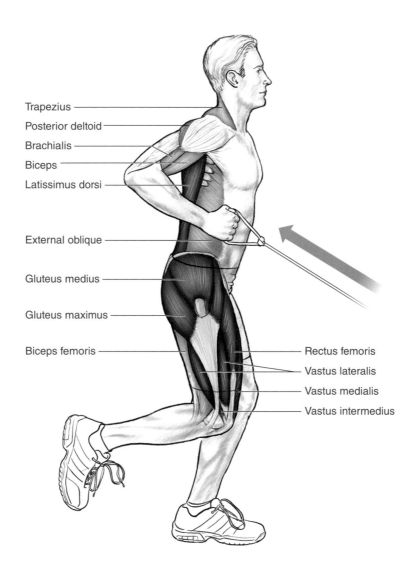

Trapezius
Posterior deltoid
Brachialis
Biceps
Latissimus dorsi

External oblique

Gluteus medius

Gluteus maximus

Biceps femoris

Rectus femoris
Vastus lateralis
Vastus medialis
Vastus intermedius

Execution

1. Balancing on one leg, face the pulley machine from about 3 to 4 feet (about 1 m) away. With an outstretched arm, grasp the stirrup handle with the opposite hand.
2. Initiating the movement with the hips, lower your body while simultaneously moving your upper extremity into a lawn-mower starting position.
3. Return to an upright position by straightening your leg and pulling the handle toward your body.
4. When pulling the handle toward your body, emphasize pinching the shoulder blade backward.

Muscles Involved

Primary: Rectus femoris, vastus lateralis, vastus intermedius, vastus medialis, gluteus maximus, gluteus medius, latissimus dorsi

Secondary: Biceps femoris, semitendinosus, semimembranosus, erector spinae, external oblique, internal oblique, trapezius, rhomboid major, rhomboid minor, teres major, posterior deltoid, biceps brachii, brachialis

Swimming Focus

By linking the movements of the upper and lower extremities and incorporating trunk rotational movements, this exercise strengthens the linkage between the arms and legs during freestyle and backstroke. Emphasizing shoulder retraction at the end of the exercise will transfer to the initial recovery process during freestyle.

To enhance the linkage between the arms and legs, setting the core at the start of the exercise is crucial. Doing this engages the core-stabilizing musculature. When performing the exercise, you should perform the movements of the upper and lower extremities in unison; separating the movements will decrease the cross-linking benefits. As with other exercises involving the lower extremity, when dropping down, the front of the knee should not extend past the tip of the toes.

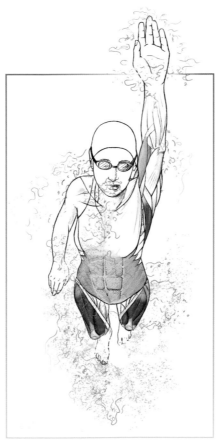

Burpee

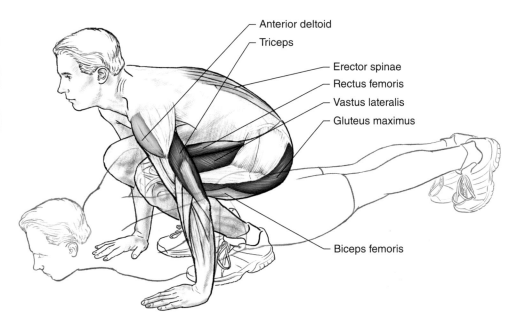

Anterior deltoid
Triceps
Erector spinae
Rectus femoris
Vastus lateralis
Gluteus maximus
Biceps femoris

Execution

1. From a standing position, drop down onto your hands and kick your feet straight back.

2. Lower into a push-up and push back up. As you complete the push-up, draw your feet forward so that they are under your hips.

3. Jump upward, lifting your arms overhead into a streamline.

4. Absorb the landing by dropping straight down into another repetition.

Muscles Involved

Primary: Rectus femoris, vastus lateralis, vastus intermedius, vastus medialis, gluteus maximus, pectoralis major, triceps brachii

Secondary: Biceps femoris, semitendinosus, semimembranosus, erector spinae, anterior deltoid

Swimming Focus

This excellent dryland exercise can be easily incorporated into a circuit-training program because no equipment is required. The primary focus of the exercise is the transition from the push-up position into the streamlined position. Emphasizing quickness when drawing the feet up under the hips will improve your speed with the open turns performed during butterfly and breaststroke. Jumping into a tight streamlined position will transfer to improved streamlining off the turn walls for all strokes.

As with regular push-ups, holding a tight body position is important; you should be able to draw a straight line from the ankles, through the hips, to the tip of the head. Sagging or arching of the low back is a technique flaw that can lead to undue stress on the spine. To protect the body, particularly the knees, from excessive pounding, you should land from the jump with the knees slightly bent to absorb the landing. Performing the exercise on a nonslip exercise mat will help protect the lower extremities from excessive pounding.

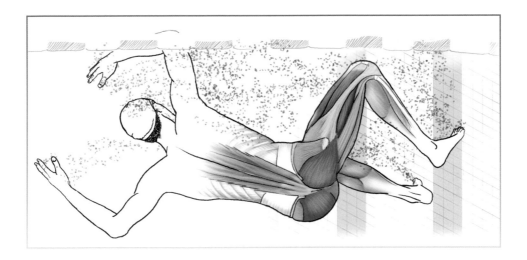

⚠ **SAFETY TIP** Before incorporating this exercise into the dryland program for a young swimmer, he or she should demonstrate the strength and coordination to perform a push-up properly.

Block Jump Start Into Streamlined Position

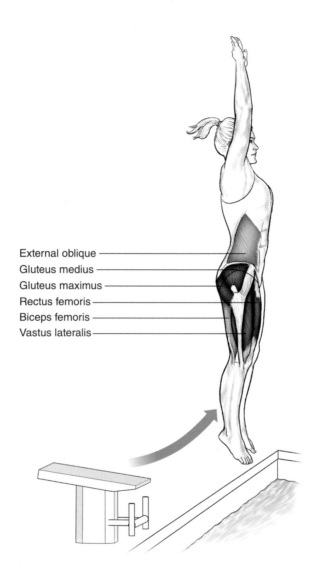

External oblique
Gluteus medius
Gluteus maximus
Rectus femoris
Biceps femoris
Vastus lateralis

Execution

1. Set yourself with your preferred starting position on the block.
2. Explode off the block into a vertical streamlined position.
3. Hold the vertical streamlined position until you enter the water.

Muscles Involved

Primary: Rectus femoris, vastus medialis, vastus intermedius, vastus lateralis, gluteus maximus, gluteus medius, erector spinae

Secondary: Biceps femoris, semitendinosus, semimembranosus, gracilis, external oblique, internal oblique, transversus abdominis

Swimming Focus

This transitional exercise helps you focus on exploding off the starting blocks into a tight streamlined position. As you jump from the blocks, the initial focus should be on jumping for maximal height. The focus then quickly shifts to holding the tight, vertical streamline. A reaction drill component can be added to the exercise by having you jump on cue.

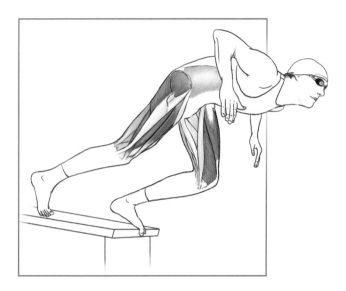

⚠ **SAFETY TIP** For safety reasons, the exercise should be performed only where the pool is at least 5 feet (150 cm) deep. The depth of the pool will dictate how long the swimmer should hold the streamlined position. For shallower pools, the swimmer should break the streamline by slightly bending the knees on entry into the water to absorb the landing when reaching the bottom of the pool. With deeper pools, the streamline can be held longer, ideally until the entire body has entered the water.

VARIATION

Dryland Block Jump Start Into Streamlined Position

The dryland variation can be used to incorporate the exercise into a circuit program or a lifting program in a weight-room environment. To avoid placing undue stress on the joints of the lower extremity, the knees should be slightly bent to absorb the landing when initially contacting the ground.

Band-Resisted Start

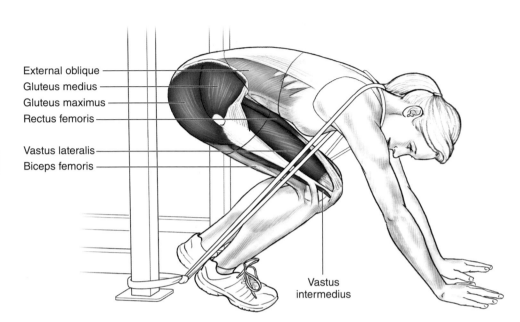

External oblique
Gluteus medius
Gluteus maximus
Rectus femoris
Vastus lateralis
Biceps femoris

Vastus intermedius

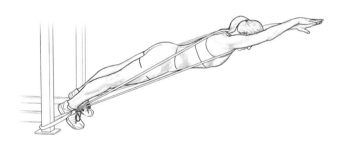

Finish position.

Execution

1. In a flat start position, set your toes and the balls of your feet against a stable object.
2. The exercise bands are brought diagonally across your body and anchored on the shoulder opposite their point of attachment.
3. Mimicking a start off the blocks, explode against the resistance of the bands.
4. To avoid reaching your arms out to catch yourself, you can bring a foot forward at end of the exercise.

Muscles Involved

Primary: Rectus femoris, vastus medialis, vastus intermedius, vastus lateralis, gluteus maximus, gluteus medius, erector spinae

Secondary: Biceps femoris, semitendinosus, semimembranosus, adductor magnus, adductor longus, adductor brevis, pectineus, gracilis, external oblique, internal oblique, transversus abdominis

Swimming Focus

This exercise specifically targets the muscles that you use to explode off the starting blocks. The key to maximizing the benefit of the exercise is to position the exercise bands so that in the starting position a small amount of tension is already placed on the bands. This tension ensures that the increased resistance and strengthening benefits will occur throughout the entire movement.

To make the exercise as realistic as possible, you should focus on transitioning into a streamlined position, just as you would during a regular start. To protect your back, set the core-stabilizing musculature at the start of the exercise and hold it tight during the entire movement. After forward movement ends, you can bring a foot forward to stabilize the body. Reaching out and then falling on an outstretched hand is a common cause of injury to the upper extremity.

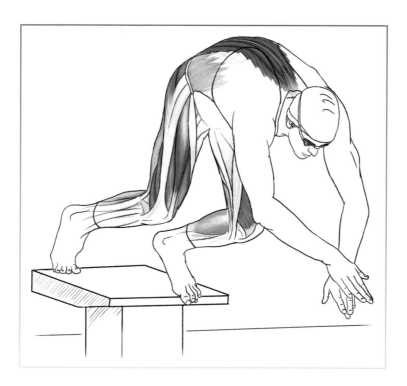

⚠️ **SAFETY TIP** Because of the complexity of this exercise, younger swimmers should **not** perform it.

Box Jump

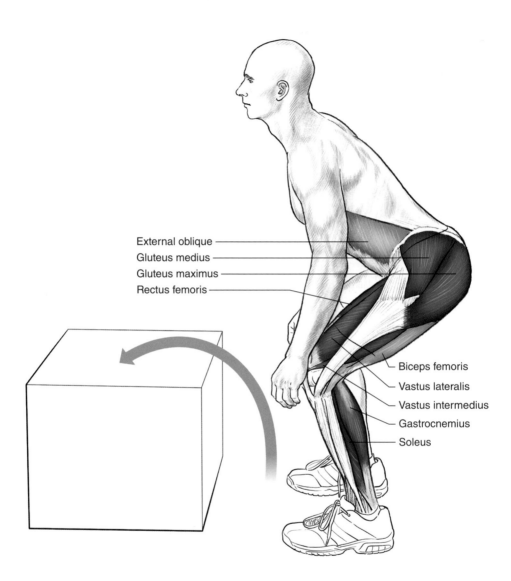

External oblique
Gluteus medius
Gluteus maximus
Rectus femoris

Biceps femoris
Vastus lateralis
Vastus intermedius
Gastrocnemius
Soleus

Execution

1. Stand 6 to 8 inches (15 to 20 cm) in front of a plyometric box and drop into a quarter-squat position.
2. Jump up onto the box, landing with your feet directly underneath you and your knees slightly flexed.
3. Complete the movement by standing up erect on the box.
4. Step off the box in a slow, controlled manner.

Muscles Involved

Primary: Rectus femoris, vastus medialis, vastus intermedius, vastus lateralis, gluteus maximus, gluteus medius, gastrocnemius, soleus

Secondary: Biceps femoris, semitendinosus, semimembranosus, external oblique, internal oblique, transversus abdominis, erector spinae

Swimming Focus

Box jumps are a valuable exercise for developing speed and strength in the lower extremities to improve your ability to explode off the starting blocks and turn walls. Jumping up onto the box has two primary advantages when compared with a normal jump for height: (1) The height of the box serves as a motivational target, and (2) landing on the box reduces the stress placed on the lower extremities. The box jump also serves as a good exercise for learning how to use the arms to increase the jump height, which translates into improved distance and speed off the starting blocks. You can increase jump height by explosively swinging the arms at the initiation of the jump.

Two common flaws associated with the exercise are tucking the legs to the chest instead of truly jumping up in the air and not keeping the chest up.

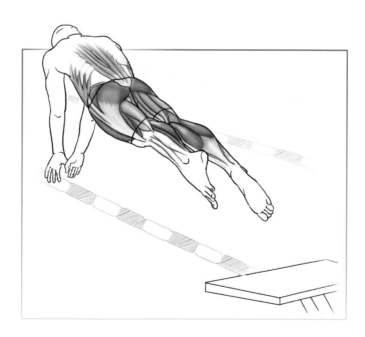

⚠ **SAFETY TIP** To avoid placing undue stress on the lower extremity, step down softly off the box instead of jumping down.

Diagonal Cable Column Lift

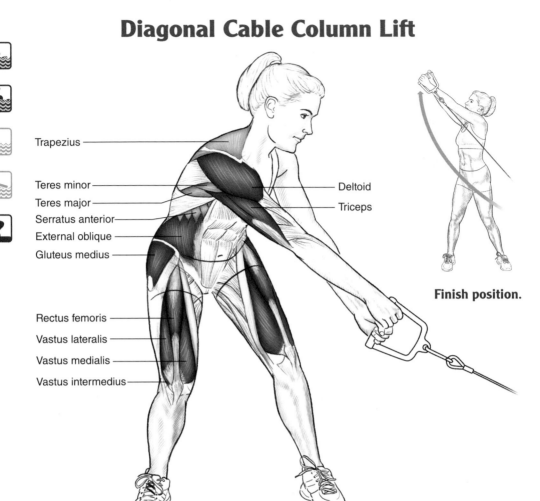

Trapezius

Teres minor
Teres major
Serratus anterior
External oblique
Gluteus medius

Rectus femoris
Vastus lateralis
Vastus medialis
Vastus intermedius

Deltoid
Triceps

Finish position.

Execution

1. Stand 2 feet (60 cm) to the side of a cable pulley machine and place your feet shoulder-width apart.
2. Drop into a half-squat and reach down and across your body to grasp the pulley handle.
3. In a combined movement, straighten your legs and pull the handle in an arcing motion up above the outer shoulder.
4. Slowly return to the starting position.

Muscles Involved

Primary: Rectus femoris, vastus medialis, vastus intermedius, vastus lateralis, gluteus maximus, gluteus medius, erector spinae, external oblique, internal oblique, anterior deltoid, middle deltoid, posterior deltoid, triceps brachii

Secondary: Biceps femoris, semitendinosus, semimembranosus, serratus anterior, trapezius, teres major, teres minor, supraspinatus, rhomboid major, rhomboid minor

Swimming Focus

The overhead reaching component of the exercise helps swimmers, particularly backstrokers, develop confidence and strength when initiating their stroke. The combined diagonal and rotational movements make this a good exercise for strengthening the core musculature while at the same time enhancing the linkage between the upper extremity and lower extremity. The leg component helps all swimmers improve their strength during starts and turns. Backstrokers will find the exercise particularly useful because it is a dryland exercise that allows them to focus on linking the movements of their arms and legs in a manner similar to that used in performing a start off the wall.

Added emphasis can be placed on the legs by deepening the squat at the start of the exercise. As with other lower-extremity exercises, be sure that the knee does not translate past the tips of the toes. To incorporate the trunk rotational movement, visually focus on following the path of the hands while performing the entire movement.

A good way to introduce this exercise to young swimmers is to begin with no resistance and later use a low-weight medicine ball.

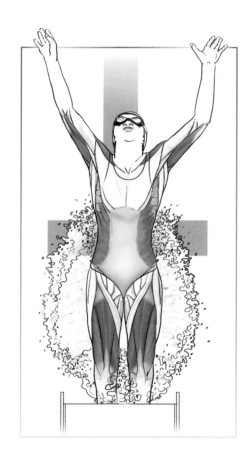

VARIATION

Diagonal Medicine Ball Lift

Using the medicine ball for resistance allows you to add an explosive component to the exercise. When performing the movement pattern with a medicine ball, emphasize throwing the medicine ball up and over one shoulder, focusing on reaching high over the shoulder.

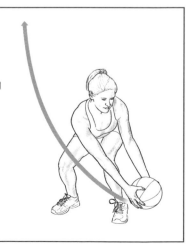

EXERCISE FINDER

ARMS

SHOULDERS

CHEST

ABDOMEN

BACK

LEGS

WHOLE BODY

ABOUT THE AUTHOR

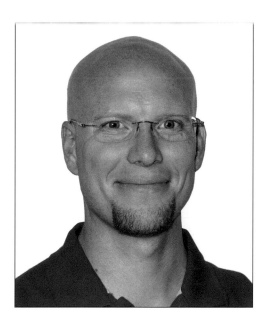

USA Swimming, the largest swimming organization in the world, specifically recommended Ian McLeod as the author of *Swimming Anatomy*. McLeod has extensive experience working with world-class athletes, particularly swimmers. A certified athletic trainer and certified massage therapist, he was a member of the U.S. team's medical staff at the 2008 Summer Olympic Games in Beijing. He has also worked extensively as an athletic trainer with the sports programs at the University of Virginia and Arizona State University.

McLeod remains deeply involved with USA Swimming's High Performance Network, a group of volunteer health professionals who support U.S. swimmers at national and international meets. He has been given the organization's highest honor, the Gold Standard Award. McLeod also served as massage therapist to the Egyptian national swim team during the 2004 Summer Olympic Games in Athens. He has provided athletic training and sport massage to swimming stars such as Ed Moses, Kaitlin Sandeno, Natalie Coughlin, and Jason Lezak.

McLeod lives in Tempe, Arizona, with his wife and two children.

ANATOMY SERIES

Each book in the *Anatomy Series* provides detailed, full-color anatomical illustrations of the muscles in action and step-by-step instructions that detail perfect technique and form for each pose, exercise, movement, stretch, and stroke.

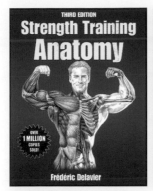

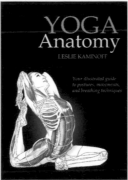

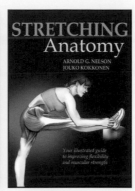

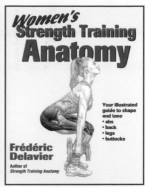

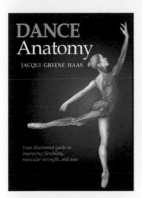

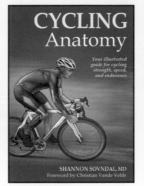

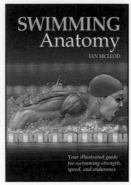

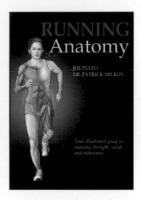

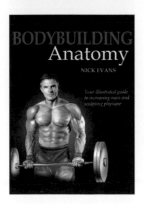

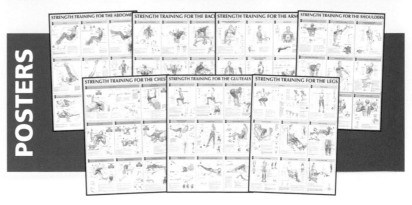

POSTERS

To place your order, U.S. customers call TOLL FREE **1-800-747-4457**
In Canada call 1-800-465-7301 • In Europe call +44 (0) 113 255 5665 • In Australia call 08 8372 0999
In New Zealand call 0800 222 062 • or visit **www.HumanKinetics.com/Anatomy**

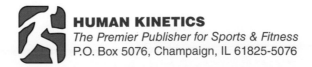

HUMAN KINETICS
The Premier Publisher for Sports & Fitness
P.O. Box 5076, Champaign, IL 61825-5076